Hepatitis B and C

Edited by Luis Rodrigo

Published in London, United Kingdom

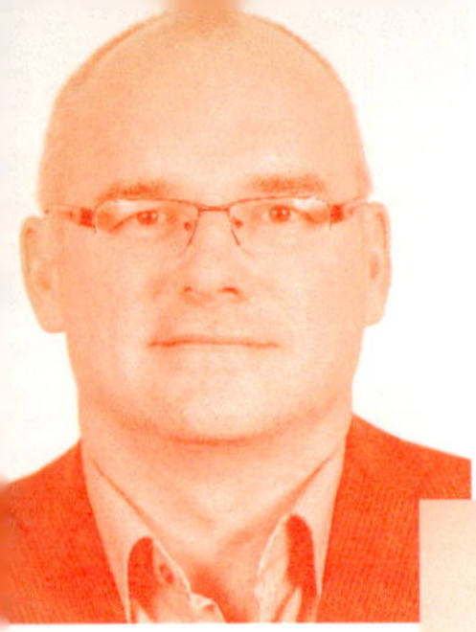
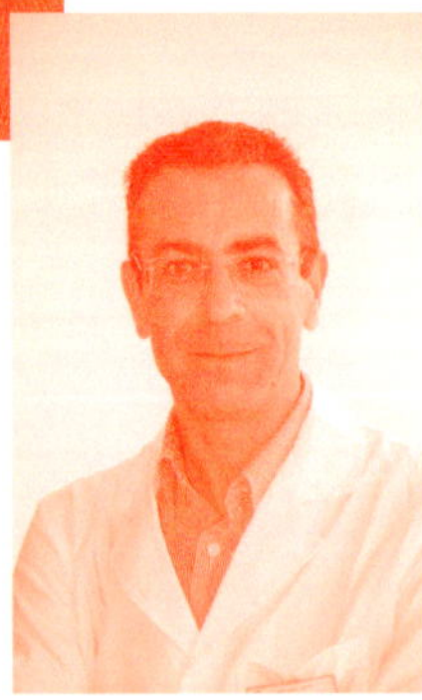
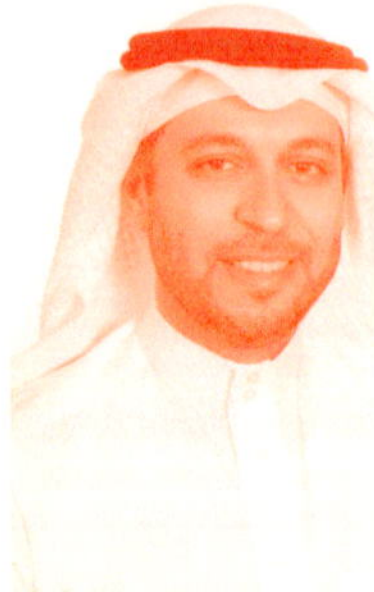
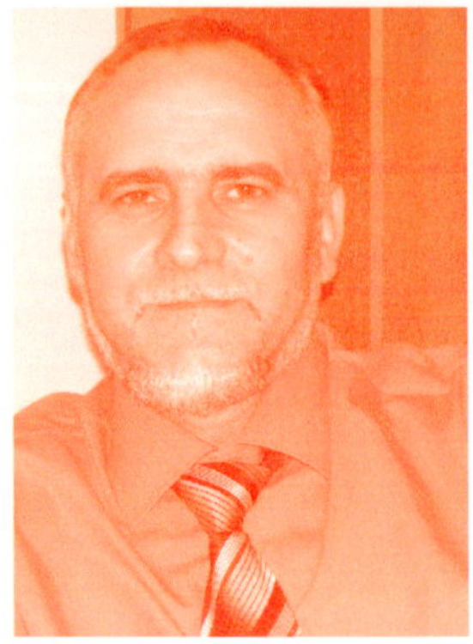
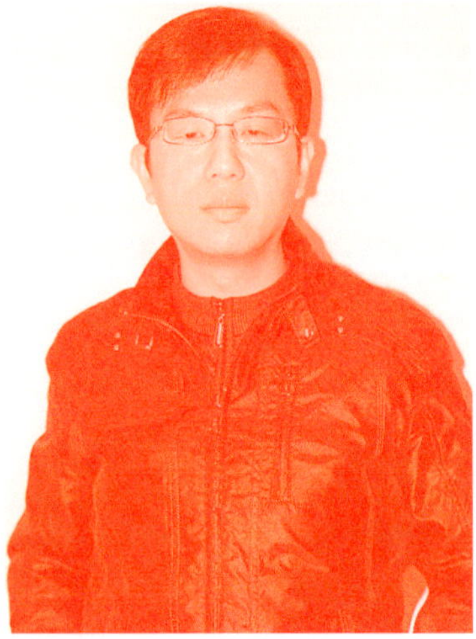
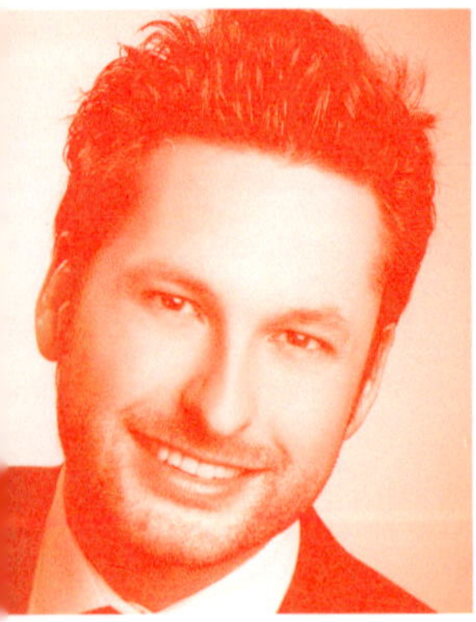
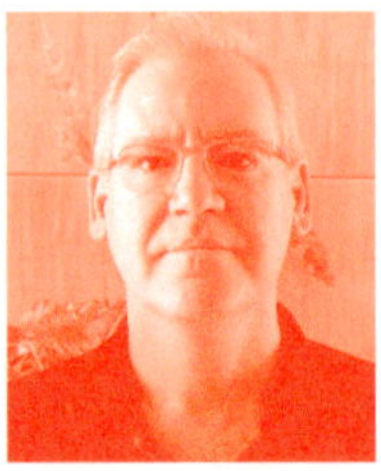

IntechOpen

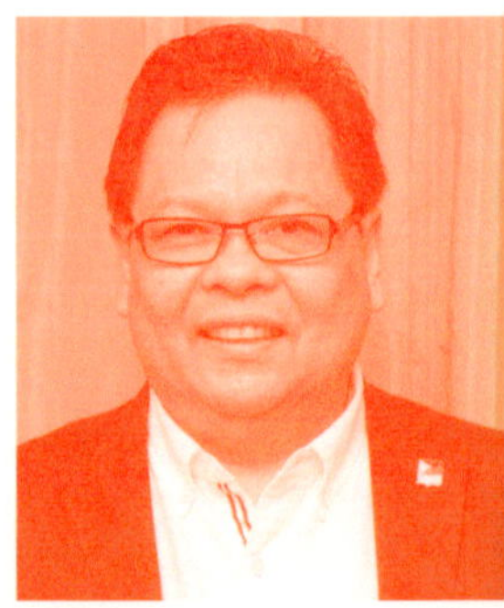
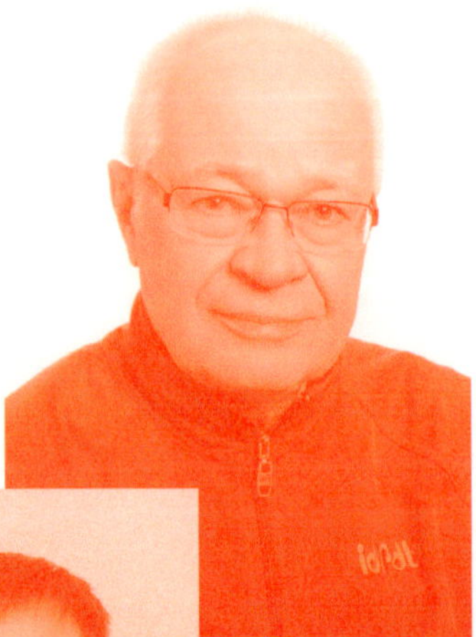
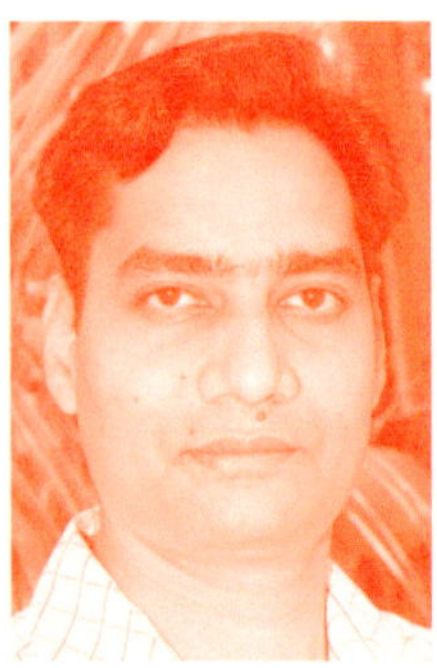
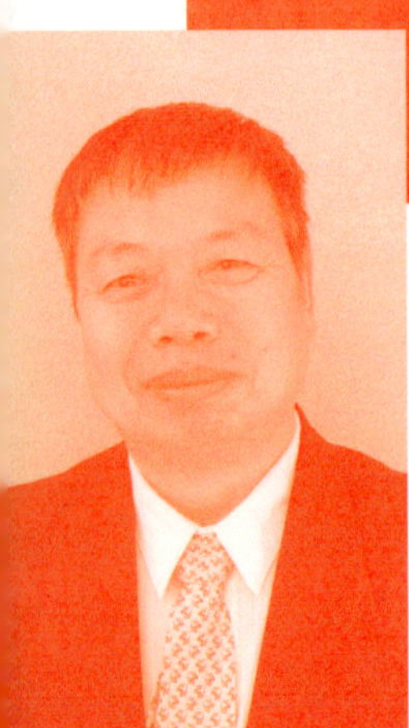
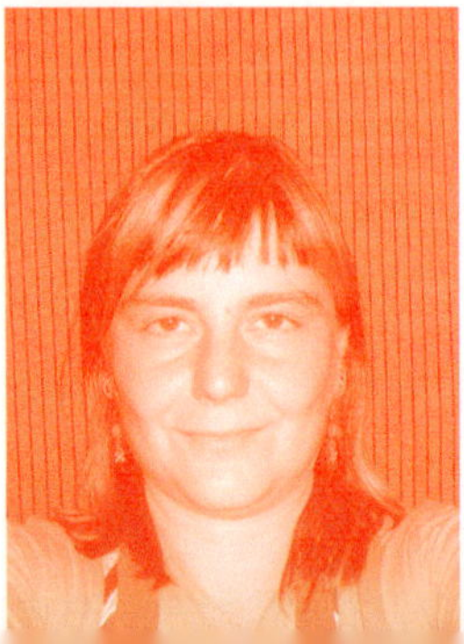
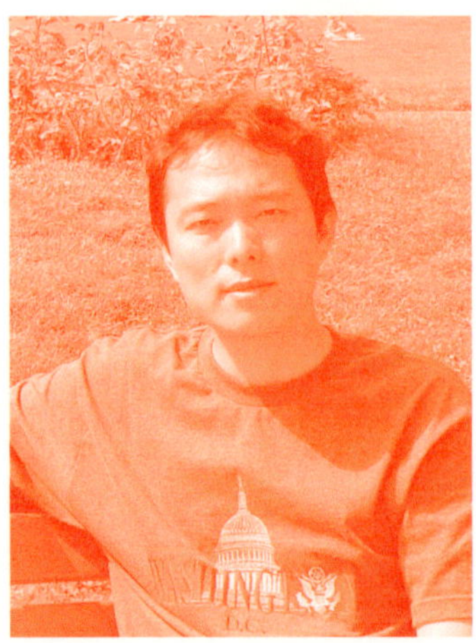

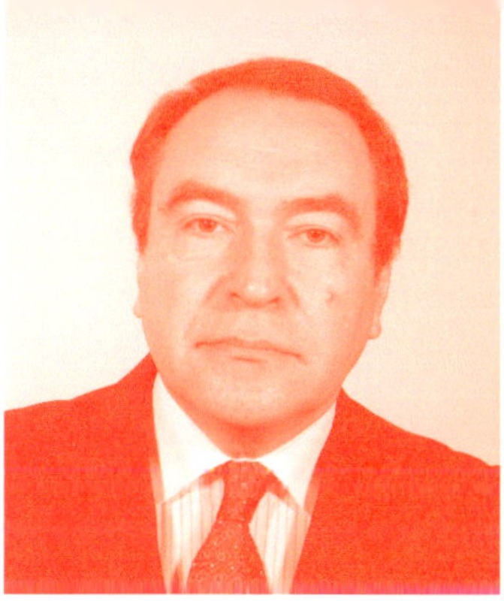
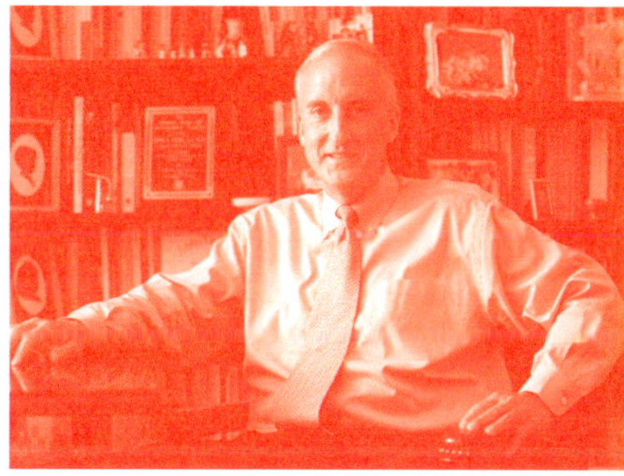
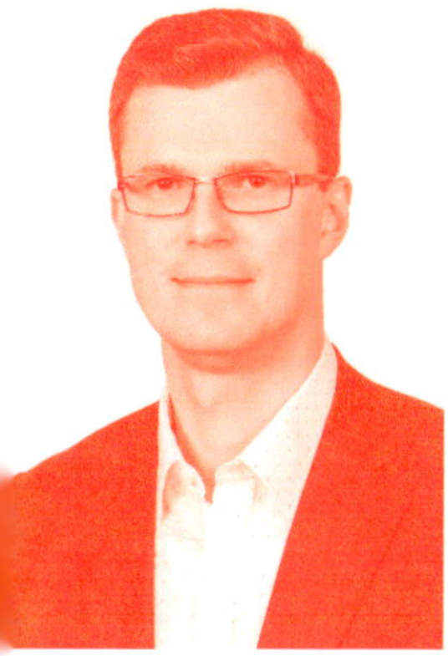
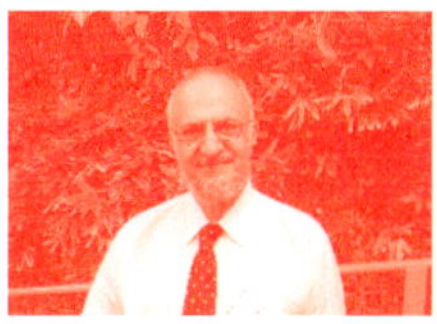
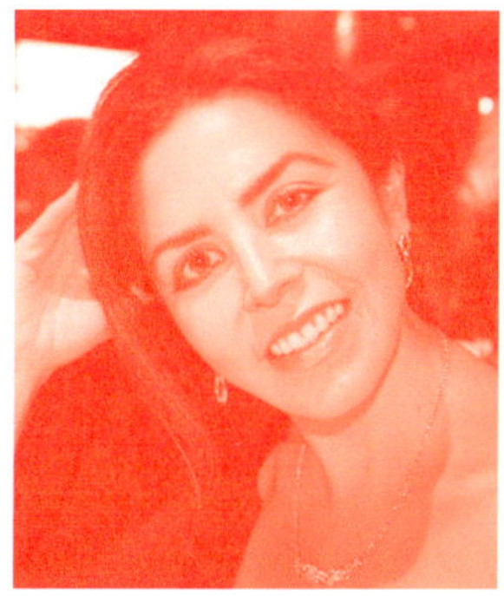

Supporting open minds since 2005

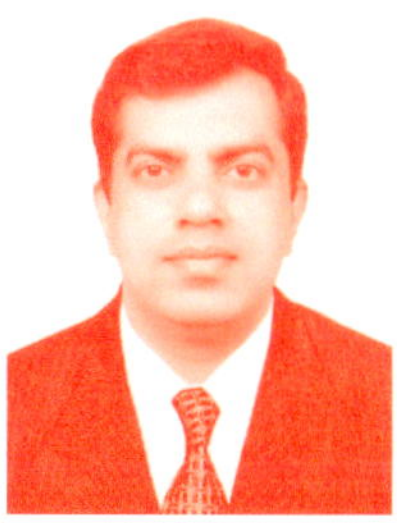
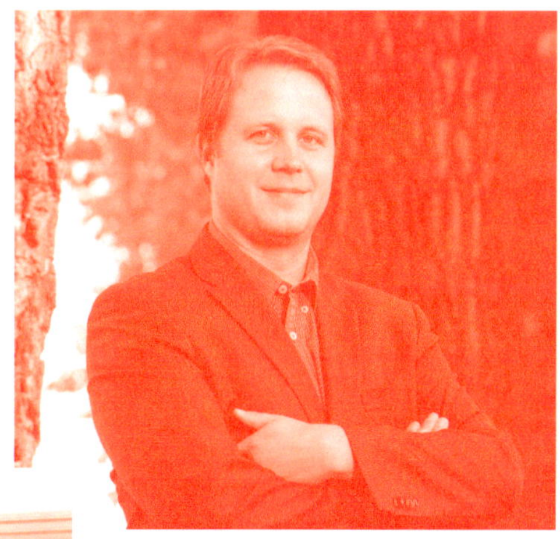
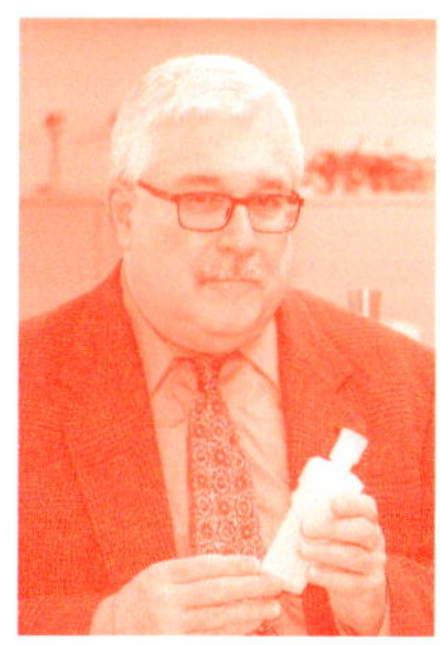
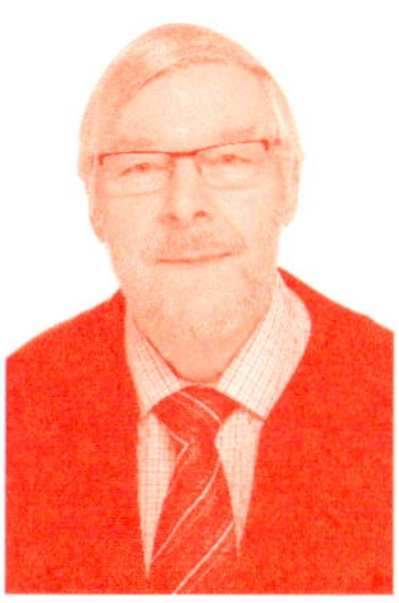
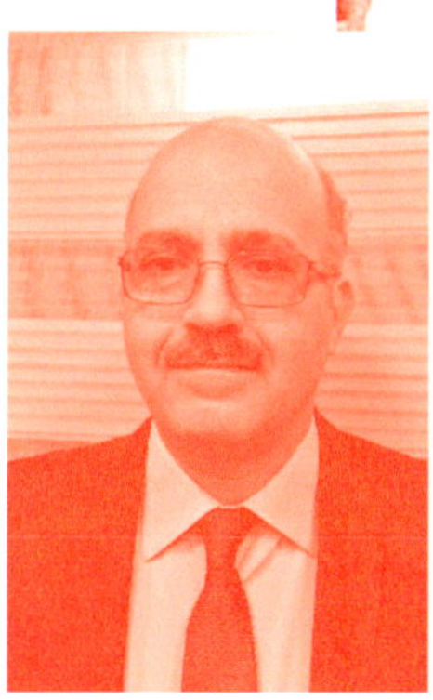
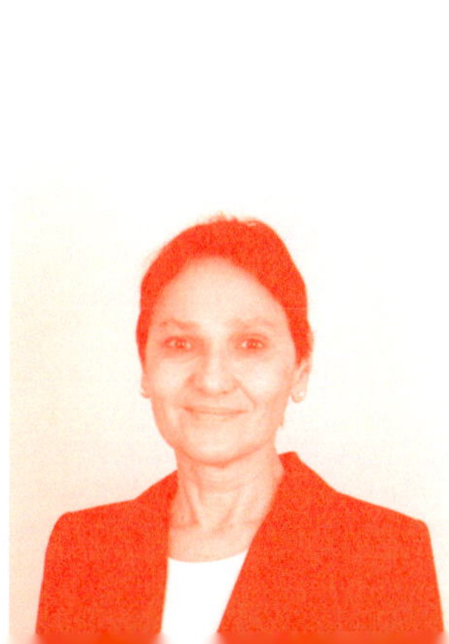
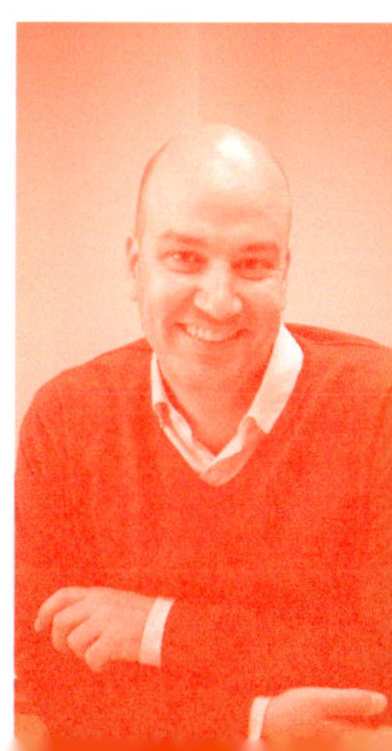

Hepatitis B and C
http://dx.doi.org/10.5772/intechopen.77706
Edited by Luis Rodrigo

Part of IntechOpen Book Series: Infectious Diseases, Volume 5
Book Series Editor: Shailendra K. Saxena

Contributors
Vijay Gayam, Smruti Mohanty, Pavani Garlapati, Arshpal Gill, Alexandra Porras-Ramírez, Alejandro Rico-Mendoza, David Kershenobich, Nayelli Flores, Damodar Paudel, Sushma Suvedi, Isaac Thom Shawa, Johra Khan

First published in London, United Kingdom, 2020 by IntechOpen
IntechOpen is the global imprint of INTECHOPEN LIMITED, registered in England and Wales, registration number: 11086078, 7th floor, 10 Lower Thames Street, London, EC3R 6AF, United Kingdom
Printed in Croatia

British Library Cataloguing-in-Publication Data
A catalogue record for this book is available from the British Library

Additional hard and PDF copies can be obtained from orders@intechopen.com

Hepatitis B and C
Edited by Luis Rodrigo
p. cm.
Print ISBN 978-1-78923-947-8
Online ISBN 978-1-78923-948-5
eBook (PDF) ISBN 978-1-83880-373-5
ISSN 2631-6188

For EU product safety concerns:
IN TECH d.o.o., Prolaz Marije Krucifikse Kozulić 3, 51000 Rijeka, Croatia,
info@intechopen.com or visit our website at intechopen.com.

IntechOpen Book Series

Infectious Diseases

Volume 5

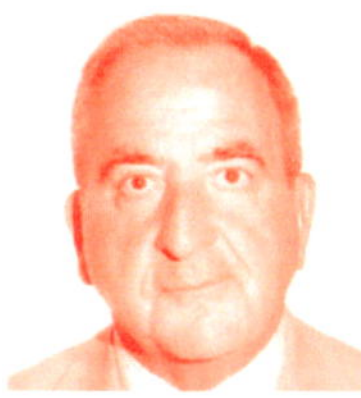

Dr Luis Rodrigo MD is an Emeritus Professor of Medicine at the University of Oviedo (Spain). He has been the Chief of Gastroenterology Service at the HUCA Hospital in Oviedo for more than 40 years. He obtained his PhD in 1975 and has a long teaching and research career. He has published a total of 590 scientific papers, 310 written in English and the rest in Spanish. He has participated as the main investigator in a total of 45 clinical trials and has directed 40 doctoral theses. He has contributed actively to the formation of around one hundred specialists in gastroenterology working in his hospital and other hospitals in Spain and abroad. He has written around 35 chapters in books of several subjects and has been the editor of 24 books in his specialty and related diseases. His areas of interest are mainly related to celiac disease and autoimmune associated diseases.

Editor of Volume 5:
Prof. Luis Rodrigo MD
Emeritus Professor of Medicine
University of Oviedo, Oviedo. Spain

Book Series Editor:
Shailendra K. Saxena
King George's Medical University

Scope of the Series

The series will give a most comprehensive overview of recent trends in various infectious diseases (as per the most recent Baltimore classification), as well as general concepts of infections, immunopathology, diagnosis, treatment, epidemiology and etiology to current clinical recommendations in management of infectious diseases, highlighting the ongoing issues, recent advances, with future directions in diagnostic approaches and therapeutic strategies. This book series will focus on various aspects and properties of infectious diseases whose deep understanding is very important for safeguarding human race from more loss of resources and economies due to pathogens.

Contents

Preface

Hepatitis B:

Viral hepatitides are important public health problems in humans. The etiologic agents were not identified until 1965, when Baruch S. Blumberg found the relationship of an Australia antigen to serum hepatitis. The antigen was found to be the surface antigen of the hepatitis B virus (HBV). This observation launched a new era in the diagnosis, prevention, and treatment of hepatitis B. Over 15 to 20 years, the natural history of HBV infection was elucidated, and more importantly, an effective vaccine became available. The routes of transmission were also made clear, rendering effective interruption in the transmission. The vaccine, together with effective interruption of the transmission, contributed greatly to the control of HBV infection. However, these measures do very little for those who have already been chronically infected. Fortunately, specific therapies against chronic hepatitis B started to appear about 10–15 years before, and the treatments have improved substantially in the last few years.

Nevertheless, hepatitis B virus infection remains a major problem for public health worldwide and represents a challenging disease for practicing physicians. Of the 2 billion people who have been infected with the hepatitis B virus, more than 350 million have chronic infections. Roughly, around 30% of the world's population show serological evidence of current or past infection. These chronically infected individuals are at high risk of death from cirrhosis and liver cancer. The use of new antiviral drugs, such us nucleotide analogues, offers hope in the prognosis of patients suffering from chronic hepatitis B.

The hepatitis B virus is a partly double-stranded DNA virus, with several serological markers: HBsAg and anti-HBs, HBeAg and anti-HBe, and anti-HBc IgM and IgG. It is transmitted through contact with infected blood and semen. A safe and effective vaccine has been available since 1981, and although variable, the implementation of universal vaccination in infants has resulted in a sharp decline in prevalence.

Hepatitis B virus is not cytopathic; both liver damage and viral control, and therefore clinical outcomes depend on the complex interplay between virus replication and host immune response. Overall, as much as 40% of men and 15% of women, with perinatally acquired hepatitis B virus infection, will die of liver cirrhosis or hepatocellular carcinoma. In addition to decreasing hepatic inflammation, long-term antiviral treatment can reverse cirrhosis and reduce hepatocellular carcinoma. Development of new therapies that can improve HBsAg clearance and virological cure is warranted.

The diffusion of HBV infection is still wide in several low-income countries, where the prevention, management, and treatment of HBV infection are a heavy burden for the governments and healthcare authorities. Of note, the information on the HBV epidemiology is minimal in numerous eastern European and Latin-American countries. The studies on molecular epidemiology performed in some countries provide an important contribution for a more comprehensive knowledge of HBV epidemiology, and phylogenetic studies provide information on the impact of recent and older migratory flows.

Occult hepatitis B virus (HBV) infection (OBI) is characterized by the persistence of HBV DNA in the liver tissue, in individuals negative for the HBV surface antigen. The prevalence of OBI is quite variable depending on the level of endemic disease in different parts of the world, the different assays utilized in the studies, and the different populations studied. Many studies have been carried out on OBI prevalence in different areas of the world and categories of individuals. The studies show that OBI prevalence seems to be higher among subjects at high risk for HBV infection and with liver disease than among individuals at low risk of infection and without liver disease.

Although far from perfect, effective means to treat those who are chronically infected now exist. In Taiwan, acute and chronic liver diseases were rampant as early as the beginning of the last century. Studies around 1975 showed an extremely high prevalence of chronic hepatitis B infection in the general population (15–20%), and 80–90% of the chronic liver diseases and hepatocellular carcinoma were caused by chronic infection with the HBV. This important health problem caught the attention of the government in the late 1970s, and a government-sponsored control program was finalized in 1981. Accordingly, a mass vaccination program against hepatitis B, primarily aiming at immunizing newborn infants, was launched on July 1, 1984. Twenty years after implementation of the program, the hepatitis B carrier rate in children covered by the program decreased by 85%, from ~15% to <1%. Most importantly, the deadly sequela of hepatocellular carcinoma in the vaccinees was also found to decrease in parallel. This is the first time that a human cancer was prevented by vaccination. Despite the success, there are still some who were born after implementation of the program but were not prevented from developing chronic hepatitis B infection and hepatocellular carcinoma. Non-compliance to the vaccination schedule, breakthrough infection, and intrauterine infection are the causes of the failure. At present, we have effective measures for immunizing susceptible individuals, interrupting the routes of transmission, and treating the chronically infected. The time for considering the elimination or even the eradication of HBV infection has come. This is especially true for countries where hepatitis B infection is not endemic. Nevertheless, with the admirable results achieved in the past, Taiwan should also think about elimination/eradication of hepatitis B, even though it will certainly be much more difficult than in the non-endemic countries.

Hepatitis C:

Hepatitis C virus (HCV) infection is a major health problem worldwide. Approximately 170–200 million individuals are chronically infected worldwide and a quarter of these patients are at increased risk of developing liver cirrhosis, hepatocellular carcinoma, and even liver failure. Cloning of the hepatitis C virus was reported in 1989. By now, the entire viral genome has been sequenced. It consists of a single-stranded positive RNA, with relationship to the Flaviviridae. The envelope region shows considerable variability. Six major genotypes have been described. HCV is transmitted via the parenteral route, mainly blood, rarely by sexual contact. Hepatitis C occurs worldwide and is found in 0.01 to 1.5% of blood donors. The immune response is unable to clear the virus in 80% of infected subjects, probably because of the hypervariability. In the acute phase the hepatitis has only mild symptoms and the chronic hepatitis usually also runs a mild course. After many years, liver cirrhosis may develop in 20% of cases; in these subjects there is a high incidence of hepatocellular carcinoma. The diagnosis can be made by detection of anti-HCV antibodies in the blood and an immunoblot confirmation test. The viral genome can be detected by the HCV-RNA (PCR) test. Immunization against hepatitis C is not possible yet.

Infection with the hepatitis C virus is an example of translational research success. The reciprocal interactions between clinicians and scientists have allowed in 30 years the initiation of empirical treatments by interferon, the discovery of the virus, the development of serological and virological tools for diagnosis but also for prognosis (the non-invasive biochemical or morphological fibrosis tests, the predictors of the specific immune response including genetic IL28B polymorphisms). Finally, well-tolerated and effective treatments with oral antivirals inhibiting HCV non-structural viral proteins involved in viral replication have been marketed this last decade, allowing for the cure of all infected subjects. HCV chronic infection, which is a public health issue, is a hepatic disease, which may lead to cirrhosis and hepatocellular carcinoma (HCC) but also a systemic disease with extra-hepatic manifestations either associated with a cryoglobulinemic vasculitis or chronic inflammation. The HCV infection is the only chronic viral infection that may be cured: the so-called sustained virologic response, defined by undetectable HCV RNA 12 weeks after the end of the treatment, significantly reduces the risk of morbidity and mortality associated with hepatic and extra-hepatic manifestations, which are mainly reversible. The history of HCV ends with the pangenotypic efficacy of multiple combinations, easy to use for 8–12 weeks with one to three pills per day and minimal intolerance issues. This explains the short 30 years from the virus discovery to the viral hepatitis elimination policy proposed by the World Health Organization (WHO) in 2016.

A complete eradication of the virus is one of the most important treatment goals for antiviral research. In 2011, the first-generation protease inhibitors boceprevir (BOC) telaprevir (TVR) was approved by FDA as the direct-acting antiviral agents. A number of promising new direct-acting antiviral agents (DAAs) have been developed in the past few years. Due to their increased efficacy, safety, and tolerability, interferon-free oral therapies with DAAs are in use for patients with chronic HCV and cirrhosis. In this review, we will discuss the results of clinical trials of several DAAs and the approved combinations, including NS3/4A protease inhibitors, NS5A inhibitors, and NS5B inhibitors. A number of drugs, including Sovaldi®, Harvoni®, Viekira Pak®, Epclusa®, Zepatier® have been approved by FDA in the last years.

Hepatitis C virus infection is a significant health problem worldwide, and is the leading cause of cirrhosis, hepatocellular carcinoma, and liver transplantation in the United States. The management of HCV has changed significantly over the last 5 years, as treatments have become simpler and more efficacious. Medication efficacy is now greater than 90%, with a high barrier to resistance and fewer side effects. This review is a collaboration between primary care and hepatology providers to explore all aspects of HCV management: acute versus chronic HCV infection, transmission and testing, and diagnosis and treatment. Specific medications for the treatment of HCV infection are considered, and patient and medication factors including genotype, liver disease status, and comorbidities affecting medication choice are discussed. This is a new era for the management of HCV infection, and interested primary care physicians, family doctors, and general internists can be at the forefront of diagnosis, management, and treatment of HCV.

DAAs have transformed traditional treatment options for hepatitis C virus infection. DAA combinations have been shown to be highly effective in reducing the burden of chronic HCV infection in clinical trials and have been recommended by the European Association for the Study of the Liver (EASL) treatment guidelines. Second generation DAAs (sofosbuvir plus daclatasvir, sofosbuvir/ledipasvir, ombitasvir/paritaprevir/ritonavir plus dasabuvir, sofosbuvir plus velpatasvir, glecaprevir plus pibrentasvir, grazoprevir plus elbasvir) have very high sustained viral response (SVR) rates and good safety profiles, higher resistance barriers, and are more convenient. Real-world data in all 3 genotypes generally support the EASL guidelines and high overall sustained virological response rates are reported with recommended regimens. However, real-world data are only available for sofosbuvir plus daclatasvir, sofosbuvir/ledipasvir, ombitasvir/paritaprevir/ritonavir plus dasabuvir. Furthermore, because of the existing level of evidence, it is difficult to define optimal regimens based on real-world data (ie, treatment duration, when to include ribavirin, and options for patients with cirrhosis). The real-life challenges of managing HIV-coinfected patients are also discussed showing the additional burden of avoiding drug-drug interactions between DAAs and antiretrovirals.

The elimination of HCV has been made possible through the availability of new antiviral drugs that may now be administered to all patients with HCV infection, even those with decompensated cirrhosis. The goal of the WHO is to reduce the incidence of chronic hepatitis infection from the current 6–10 million to 0.9 million cases of chronic infections by 2030, and annual deaths from 1.4 million to fewer than 0.5 million. Achieving these targets will require full implementation of epidemiological knowledge of HCV infection, screening and testing practices, and strategies to link HCV patients to care.

Prof. Luis Rodrigo, MD
Emeritus Professor of Medicine,
University of Oviedo,
Oviedo, Spain

Section 1

Hepatitis B

Chapter 1

Molecular Variants for HBsAg: Surface and Subtype

Johra Khan

Abstract

Hepatitis B is a worldwide healthcare problem, especially in developing areas. An estimated one-third of the global population has been infected with this virus; approximately 350 million people are lifelong carriers, and only 2% spontaneously seroconvert annually. Hepatitis B virus (HBV) belongs to the hepadnavirus family of enveloped DNA viruses containing a partially double-stranded genome of 3182 ± 3221 bp depending on the genotype that encodes four overlapping open reading frames. HBV is classified into eight genotypes (A–H) that are geographically dispersed. Genotype A is predominant in North America, Western Europe, and Africa; genotypes B and C in Asia; genotype D in Southern Europe, Africa, and India; genotype E in West Africa; genotype F in Central and South America and Alaska; genotype G has been found in the United States, France, and Germany; and genotype H in Central America. Genotypes A, B, C, and D predominate in the United States, while the other genotypes are less common. Further detailed analysis of these HBsAg variants would provide further understanding of the antigenic structure of HBV.

Keywords: genotypes, subtypes, surface antigen, hydrophilic region, HBsAg variants

1. Introduction

A report by Blumberg in 1965 led to the discovery of hepatitis B surface antigen (HBsAg) which is also known as Australian antigen and its related antibody which is hepatitis B surface antibody or HBsAb [1]. After a gap of 5 years, in 1970, another scientist, Dane, visualized the hepatitis B (HBV). Since that time, a significant development has been made about the epidemiology, virology, natural history, and the treatment of this hepatotropic virus. It is the smallest of the DNA viruses that infect man and cause acute hepatitis of varying severity. It is an extremely resistant strain capable of withstanding extreme temperatures and humidity. It can survive when stored for 25 years at −20°C, for 24 months at −80°C, for 6 months at room temperatures, and for 7 days at 44°C [2].

Hepatitis B is a global healthcare problem, especially found in developing countries. As per an estimate, one third of the world population has been infected with this virus which is around 350 million people are enduring carriers and only 2% of them are spontaneously seroconvert yearly [3]. Many current vaccination programs seem to be promising in the effort to reduce the incidence of this disease [4]. HBV is transmitted through hematological and sexual means. The consequence of this infection is a complex viral-host interaction which results in either as an acute disease with symptoms or an asymptomatic disease. Patients may develop an immunity to HBV or it may enter a chronic carrier state (**Figure 1**). The later consequences of this infection are cirrhosis and then development of hepatocellular carcinoma (HCC) [5]. Hepatitis B virus (HBV) belongs to the hepadnavirus family of enveloped DNA viruses containing a partially double-stranded genome of 3182 ± 3221 bp depending on the genotype which encodes four overlapping and open reading frames which are as follows:

- S for the surface or envelope gene encoding the pre-S1, pre-S2, and the S protein
- C for the core gene, encoding for the core nucleocapsid protein and the "e" antigen
- X for the X gene encoding the X protein
- P for the polymerase gene encoding, a large protein promoting priming, RNA-dependent and DNA-dependent DNA polymerase, and RNase H activities

The genome is read in all three reading frames, and viral regulatory elements are all within coding regions which introduce constraints on the ability of the virus to accept mutations and remain viable [6]. Nevertheless, heterogeneity among the strains of HBV circulating globally is 10%-fold greater than that in the majority of DNA viral genomes. This is explained, at least partially, by the fact that hepadnavirus replication takes place via an RNA intermediate, and reverse transcriptase is known to have a high error rate 16. A nucleotide exchange rate of between 0–1 and 0–7 per year [7] has been estimated for the HBV [8] and woodchuck hepatitis virus (WHV) [9]; genomes, respectively, which is similar

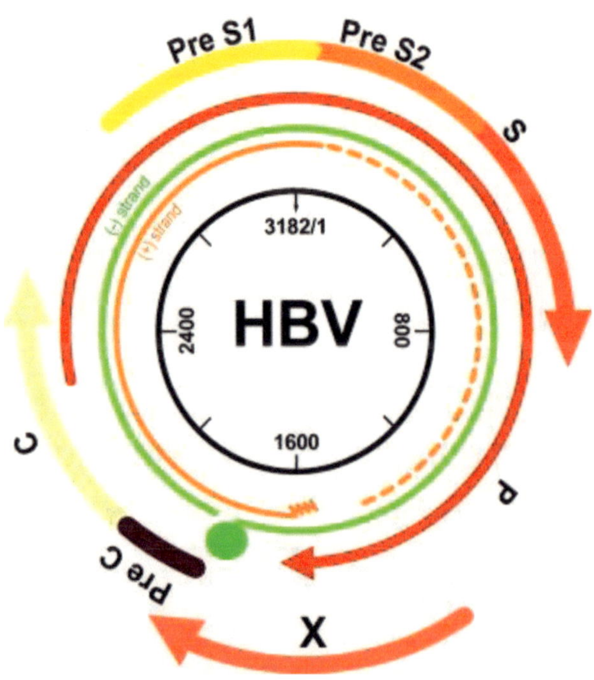

Figure 1.
HBV genome showing S for the surface or envelope gene encoding the pre-S1, pre-S2, and the S protein.

to the most slowly evolving gene of retroviruses, the gag gene, and one to two orders of magnitude lower than the mutation rates previously calculated for the positive- and negative-strand RNA viruses [10]. The virus persists in 2–10% of adult patients and approximately 90% of infected infants leading to chronic liver disease. In highly endemic areas, infection is predominantly acquired during the perinatal neonatal period or by horizontal transmission in the first few years of life [10, 11] which results in a high prevalence of long-term HBV carriers with a low average age at infection [12], the virus has a long time span in which to evolve within its host.

1.1 Natural history

Acute infection with HBV in adulthood is rarely associated with the development of potentially fatal fulminant liver failure. Chronic infection, whether acquired in childhood or in adulthood, is associated with progressive liver disease, risk of cirrhosis, liver failure, and HCC and rarely with extrahepatic manifestations. Chronic HBV infection is characterized by four distinct phases: immune tolerance, immune clearance, inactive carrier state, and reactivation [13]. The immune tolerance phase is characterized by detectable HBeAg, high levels of HBV DNA (>105 copies/ml), and normal ALT levels. The immune clearance phase, also called CHB, is characterized by detectable or undetectable HBeAg, undetectable or detectable anti-HBe antibodies, lower or fluctuating levels of HBV DNA, high or fluctuating ALT levels, and active inflammation as seen on liver biopsy. The inactive HBsAg carrier state is characterized by detectable HBsAg, undetectable HBeAg, detectable anti-HBe antibodies, low levels of HBV DNA (<104 copies/ml), and normal ALT levels. Later in the carrier phase, HBsAg may become undetectable, and anti-HBs antibodies may appear [13], although reactivation can occur in inactive HBV carriers (**Figure 2**).

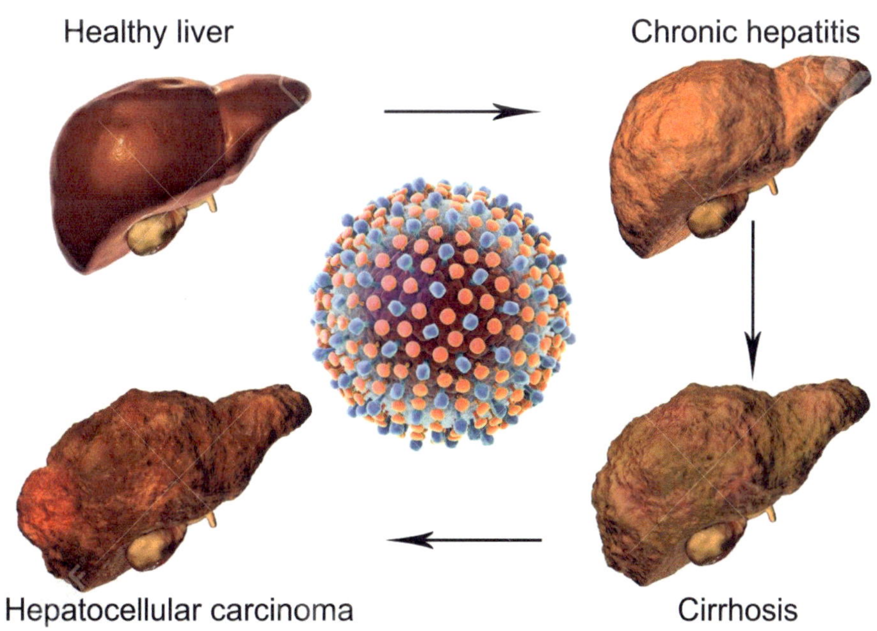

Figure 2.
Different stages of HBV infection. https: //www.123rf.com/photo_83543016_stock-illustration-liver-disease-progression-in-hepatitis-c-virus-infection-3d-illustration.html.

2. The surface gene and variants

HBV is classified into eight genotypes (A–H) that are geographically dispersed. Genotype A is predominant in North America, Western Europe, and Africa; genotypes B and C in Asia; genotype D in Southern Europe, Africa, and India; genotype E in West Africa; genotype F in Central and South America and Alaska; genotype G has been found in the United States, France, and Germany; and genotype H in Central America. Genotypes A, B, C, and D predominate in the United States, while the other genotypes are less common. 31 Genotype B is associated with less active disease, slower progression, and lower incidence of hepatocellular carcinoma (HCC) than genotype C. Genotypes A and B generally respond better to treatment with interferon than do genotypes C and D. No relation between HBV genotypes and response to nucleos(t)ide analogue-based therapies has been demonstrated 31.

Originally, four genotypic groups of HBV (A–D) were defined, based on an inter-genotypic divergence score of 8 ± 5–10 ± 0% between 18 complete genomes, as compared to a score of 1 ± 1–2 ± 7% between isolates within the same genotype [14]. This genotypic classification was extended to six genotypes (A–F) by phylogenetic analysis of 122 surface antigen (HBsAg) genes [15]. The genotypic groups are geographically arranged [16] with genotypes B and C confined to Asia, while genotype A predominates in Northern Europe giving way to genotype D as one moves toward the Mediterranean region. Genotype E is mainly found in parts of East, Central, and West Africa, and genotype F is only found in the New World and the Pacific which is also home to the Cq—subgroup of genotype C [17]. Two subgroups of genotype A, subgroups A and A, were found in approximately equal amounts in an urban population from South Africa together with 10% of genotype D [17].

In the recent advances in molecular diagnostic techniques, it was found that HBV envelop is made of host-derived bilayer of phospholipids encoded by S gene. c1.

3. The surface gene variants

The mutation in HBV depends on the high rate of replication of this virus which in turn depends on RNA- dependent DNA polymerase. In highly variant individuals, the mutation of genome can be up to 10^{10} per day. Whereas most of the variants produced are defective, some of them can cause infection or reason for treatment failure.

3.1 HBsAg variants

In the structure of virus, the coat of the outer surface is made up of hepatitis B surface proteins which are made in larger amounts than needed by the virus to its reproduction process. The excess amount of these surface proteins clusters together into some spherical units of size between 17 and 25 nm of diameter, and sometimes it also forms rods of different lengths. It is found that in some studied cases, these units condense as a core particle to produce a whole and infectious virus unit that passes into the blood stream and can also infect many other healthy liver cells. All the different structures like extra spheres, rodlike and also sometimes complete viral particles easily move in the blood stream in large amount and can be easily detected; only it takes little long time for these protein particles to appear in blood.

The incubation time for this hepatitis B Virus (hepatitis B) can be between 6 and 25 weeks. It was found that after infection for up to 1 to 6 weeks before symptoms start occurring, HBsAg appears. To confirm the presence of hepatitis B infection, the positive result for the presence of hepatitis B surface protein (HBsAg) is the available standard test to indicate current infection. If the hepatitis B surface protein (HBsAg) remains present for a time of more than 6 months, it is generally considered as an indicator for chronic infection.

It is reported that if excess of HBs proteins is produced, it may allow infectious hepatitis B virus particles to leak the immune system by mopping some low levels of surface antibodies that may be produced by the immune system due to its 145 amino acid which is glycine that changes to arginine (G145R) [18].

3.2 Hepatitis B core protein (HBcAg)

The HBc proteins link together to form the hepatitis B core that encapsulates HBV DNA and DNA polymerase; this core is in turn encapsulated by HBs proteins.

The core protein (HBc) is not detectable in the bloodstream; however it can be detected in the sample of liver cells taken after a liver biopsy.

3.3 HBe protein (HBeAg or "e" antigen)

The Hepatitis B "e" antigen (HBeAg) is a peptide and normally detectable in the bloodstream when the hepatitis B virus is actively reproducing; this in turn leads to the person being much more infectious and at a greater risk of progression to liver disease. The exact function of this nonstructural protein is unknown; however it is thought that HBe may be influential in suppressing the immune system response to HBV infection. HBeAg is generally detectable at the same time as HBsAg and disappears before HBsAg disappears. The presence of HBeAg in chronic infection is generally taken to indicate that HBV is actively reproducing and there is a higher probability of liver damage. In acute infection HBeAg is generally only transiently present [19].

However mutant strains of HBV exist that replicate without producing HBeAg. In many cases infection with these mutant strains is more aggressive than HBe producing strains [20].

4. Variants associated with antiviral therapy

Polymerase variants are another class of variants detected during therapy with nucleoside analogues which become the reason for drug resistance. The most recognized mutation affecting lamivudine drug is due to change in 204 amino acid from methionine to valine or isoleucine (M204 V/I) which sometimes occurs with another change at 180 amino acid position (L180 M). This change helps in replication and healthy survival of the mutant.

In HBV-infected patients during liver transplant therapy, antiviral prophylaxis is combined with HBIG drug as the polymerase gene and surface gene in HBV have the same regions of the genome; although read in a different frame, the mutation in one can force the other for it. This could lead to complications in selection of mutants for both HBsAg and HBV polymerase [21].

4.1 HBV variants associated with active immunization

Active immunization is the most effective way to control the prominent cause of hepatitis, human hepatitis B virus (HBV). The highly antigenic hepatitis B surface antigen (HBsAg) is directly related to induce the humoral immune response, which on the other hand provides immunity against HBV infection. Neutralizing B cell epitopes are believed to be due to changes in position 124 to 147 of HBsAg, defined as the "a" determinant [22].

In recent years, HBV variants with mutations on the “a” determinant have been recognized following vaccination. These mutants are proficient in independent replication and lead to active infection [23–25]. These mutations have been identified at various positions on the “a” determinant, the most often identified being the glycine-to-arginine change at position 145 (G145R) of HBsAg [25–31].

The most important is that some of the mutants existed before the vaccination program is introduced. These include changes of amino acids at positions 126, 129, 133, and 145 [29, 31]. Some of these are naturally occurring HBsAg variants which are transmissible and are able to infect even the vaccinated population [29, 31]. HBsAg variants have recently been recognized on the major hydrophilic loop of HBsAg (aa 100–160) but outside the conventional “a” determinant [32]. These new mutants can occur in both the vaccinated and unvaccinated individuals in a population and are not able to be neutralized by the presently available antibodies.

5. HBsAg in liver transplantation

The patients suffering with chronic HBV contagion are having high risk of developing cirrhosis and hepatic liver failure and having hepatocellular carcinoma. The well-known orthotopic liver transplantation (OLT) procedure is a well-established treatment for liver failure and other hepatocellular carcinoma patients. The occurrence of HBV infection creates many exceptional issues with patients undergoing orthotopic liver transplantation treatment. The inability to get treatment and HBV reinfection occurs in almost 75–80% of persons who undergo OLT treatment. Recurrence of HBV infection even after OLT repeatedly followed by aggressive clinical treatments and also related with a major decrease in successful graft and the rate of patient recovery. In recent times some new antiviral therapies and prophylactic schemes using hepatitis B immune globulin (HBIG) have been established to decrease the risk of recurrence of HBV infection in OLT patients.

5.1 Liver transplantation after treatment of HBV infection

There are numerous aims of providing antiviral therapy to patients with cirrhosis which is secondary to prolonged HBV infection. The patients who have with compensated cirrhosis, they can get antiviral therapy which can inhibit development to decompensated cirrhosis and eradicate the possible requirement for OLT treatment. The antiviral therapy can effectively decrease the risk of advancement to hepatocellular carcinoma.

For patients having decompensated cirrhosis, antiviral therapy can improve liver function which can also delay the need for transplantation. If the patient’s condition progresses to the point that transplantation is needed, the aim of antiviral therapy is to minimize the HBV risk at the time of transplantation, thereby controlling the risk of recurrence of HBV infection after OLT.

5.1.1 Major therapies for minimizing HBV infection or recurrence

IFN-α: Before starting treatment with IFN-α, the hazards and uses related to IFN-α therapy must be carefully assessed in patients having cirrhosis with chronic HBV infections. IFN-α treatment is related with a burst in serum aminotransferases in 35–55% of already treated patients. For patients having progressive liver disease, IFN-α rehabilitation may increase the hepatic breakdown, so it has to be avoided. IFN-α treatment can aggravate cytopenia and additional intensification the risk of severe bacterial toxicities. IFN-α treatment can be provided safely by keeping close monitoring system for the patients having compensated cirrhosis [33]. Some researchers prove that up to 31% of the cirrhotic HBV patients cured using IFN-α-2b had showed seroconversion of antibody related to hepatitis B antigen, and they lose of measureable HBV DNA, in response rates which are similar to that of the non-cirrhotic patients. Various studies had shown that the cirrhotic patients who have lost HBeAg show superior up to 10 years of survival rate in comparison to the patients who had shown no response to IFN-α therapy [34]. Some of the researchers had shown in there research that the rate of incidence of hepatocellular carcinoma may be lesser in patients who had received treatment using IFN-α, generally in the subcategory of patients who had cleared HBV DNA from their blood serum [35, 36]. Generally, the risks related to IFN-α treatment and the occurrence of harmless and well-tolerated oral antiviral therapies have reduced the usefulness of IFN-α treatment in patients having cirrhosis. Pegylated IFN-α-2a was newly accepted by the US Food and Drug Administration to be used for the treatment of chronic hepatitis B. A few related data is presently available showing the use of pegylated IFN-α in relation to cirrhotic patients having hepatitis B.

Lamivudine: It is based on nucleoside analogue which is an effective inhibitor of HBV DNA replication process. It was one of the first accepted orally administered medications to be used for the treatment of patients having chronic HBV infection. It has also confirmed an exceptional safety picture in both the compensated and uncompensated patients of cirrhosis. In patients suffering from decompensated cirrhosis because of HBV infection, lamivudine is shown to be a safe and effective drug therapy. Previous researches having uncontrolled case studies show the conflicted results for lamivudine treatment which was shown to delay advancement to death or toward liver transplantation [37, 38]. Liaw et al. [39] stated the results related to a large, potential, multicenter randomized trial based on the study of 651 patients who had chronic hepatitis B, and bridging fibrosis was randomized to obtain any of the lamivudine or placebo. The basic points of this research was time essential for the disease development, which is also known as hepatic compensation, hepatocellular carcinoma, spontaneous bacterial peritonitis, variceal bleeding, or death associated with liver disease. After they receive a treatment for a period of 32.4 months which can range from 0 to 42 months in which a substantially larger percentage of patients in the placebo group in contrast to the lamivudine group developed disease advancement (17.7% vs. 7.8%; Pp. 001), because of which the study was finished early. Moreover, hepatocellular carcinoma arose in a less percentage of patients in the lamivudine-treated individual than in the placebo group (3.9% vs. 7.4%, Pp .047). The results show that based on lamivudine is more effective in reducing the occurrence of hepatic decompensation and hepatocellular carcinoma in patients who have chronic HBV infection and also progressive fibrosis or cirrhosis. The main aspect reducing the use of lamivudine is that it causes the increase of mutations in the YMDD motif of the HBV DNA polymerase gene, which develops resistance against lamivudine. YMDD mutations are emerging with a rate of ~20% every year against lamivudine treatment which are related to the return of active viral replication [40]. The findings of lamivudine resistance in clinical setting vary according to the rigorousness of underlying liver damage. The initial sign related to resistance usually occurs as a recoil in the HBV DNA level, lacking any other irregular biochemical or clinical results. However, advanced liver failure has been defined in connotation with the occurrence of YMDD mutations.

So, patients with cirrhosis need closely observing during their receiving prolonged lamivudine therapy.

Adefovir dipivoxil: An oral prodrug of adefovir which is a nucleotide analogue of adenosine monophosphate that inhibits HBV DNA polymerase. Many studies show that adefovir has tremendous activity against wild-type as well as lamivudine-resistant HBV strains. Researchers evaluated the safety and efficacy of adefovir dipivoxil (10 mg daily) in 128 patients having lamivudine-resistant HBV and are waiting for liver transplantation. Treatment for a period of 48 weeks managed to cause an average decrease in HBV DNA titer of 4.1 log10 copies/ml, where as in non-detectable HBV DNA (by PCR; lower limit of detection, 400 copies/ml), it was in 81% and showed better Child-Pugh score which is up to 92%. Adefovir dipivoxil treatment can generally be accepted very finely with an increase in their serum creatinine level up to 10.5 mg/dL from baseline in around 12% of the patients. No patient is required to stop adefovir dipivoxil therapy due to nephrotoxicity. The survival rate after 48 weeks was 84% which is significantly better than the rate for historical control subjects.

Other oral agents: Entecavir a new guanosine nucleoside analogue which was recently accepted by the US Food and Drug Administration for the treatment of chronic hepatitis B. Although no publication is done, but a huge phase III research has proven that HBeAg-positive patients provided with entecavir (0.5 mg daily for 48 weeks) showed a mean change in HBV DNA titer of _6.98 log10 copies/ml, which was considerably better than that was found with lamivudine [33]. Entecavir has also revealed activity against lamivudine- and adefovir dipivoxil-resistant HBV strains. Still there are no exact data available on the use of entecavir in patients with decompensated cirrhosis or in association with liver transplantation.

6. Conclusion

HBsAg variants with changes outside the "a" identification of these new HBsAg variants and their functional analysis may provide further understanding of the antigenic structure of HBV; also liver transplantation for hepatitis B is having complication of the risk of recurring HBV infection. It significantly reduces the rates of graft success and patient survival after transplantation. Effective therapy with OLT recipient patients having chronic HBV infection involves management of antiviral therapy before OLT to reduce the hepatitis B viral titer at the time of transplantation.

Acknowledgements

I am grateful to Deanship of Scientific Research, Majmaah University, Al Majmaah 11952, Saudi Arabia, for providing support for this research.

Conflict of interest

I declare that there is no conflict of interest with any or all the above writing.

Author details

Johra Khan
College of Applied Medical Sciences, Department of Medical Laboratories, Majmaah University, Al Majmaah, Saudi Arabia

*Address all correspondence to: j.khan@mu.edu.sa

References

[1] Blumberg BS, Alter HJ, Visnich S. Landmark article Feb 15, 1965: A "new" antigen in leukemia sera. By Baruch S. Blumberg, Harvey J. Alter, and Sam Visnich. Journal of the American Medical Association. 1984;**252**(2):252-257

[2] Dane DS, Cameron CH, Briggs M. Virus-like particles in serum of patients with Australia-antigen-associated hepatitis. Lancet. 1970;**1**(7649):695-698

[3] Pungpapong S, Kim WR, Poterucha JJ. Natural history of hepatitis B virus infection: An update for clinicians. Mayo Clinic Proceedings. 2007;**82**(8):967-975

[4] Shen LP, Yang JY, Mo ZJ, Li RC, Li YP, Wei ZL, et al. Variations of hepatitis B virus infection epidemic pattern after long-term HBV vaccine immunization. Zhonghua Shi Yan He Lin Chuang Bing Du Xue Za Zhi. 2007;**21**(3):253-255

[5] Natural history of chronic hepatitis B virus infection in adults with emphasis on the occurrence of cirrhosis and hepatocellular carcinoma. Journal of Gastroenterology and Hepatology. 2000;**15**(Suppl):E25-E30

[6] Yang Z, Lauder IJ, Lin HJ. Molecular evolution of the hepatitis B virus genome. Journal of Molecular Evolution. 1995;**41**:587-596

[7] Boyer JC, Bebenek K, Kunkel TA. Unequal HIV-1 reverse transcriptase error rates with RNA and DNA templates. Proceedings of the National Academy of Sciences, USA. 1992;**89**:6919-6923

[8] Gunther S, Fischer L, Puli I, Sterneck M, Will H. Naturally occurring variants of hepatitis B. In: Advances in Viral Research. 1999. pp. 25-137

[9] Okamoto H, Imai M, Kametani M, Nakamura T, Mayumi M. Genomic heterogeneity of hepatitis B virus in a 54-year-old woman who contracted the infection through materno-fetal transmission. The Japanese Journal of Experimental Medicine. 1987;**57**:231-236

[10] Girones R, Miller RL. Mutation rate of the hepadnavirus genome. Virology. 1989;**170**:595-597

[11] Beasley RP, Hwang LY. Epidemiology of hepatocellular carcinoma. In: Viral Hepatitis and Liver Disease. 1984. pp. 209-224

[12] Botha JF, Dusheiko GM, Ritchie MJJ, Mouton HWK, Kew MC. Hepatitis B virus carrier state in black children in Ovamboland: Role of perinatal and horizontal infection. Lancet. 1984:1210-1212

[13] Edmunds WJ, Medley GF, Nokes DJ, O'Callaghan CJ, Whittle HC, Hall AJ. Epidemiological patterns of hepatitis B virus (HBV) in highly endemic areas. Epidemiology and Infection. 1996;**117**:313-325

[14] Yim HJ, Lok AS. Natural history of chronic hepatitis B virus infection: What we knew in 1981 and what we know in 2005. Hepatology. 2006;**43**(2 suppl 1):S173-S181

[15] Chandra R, Kapoor D, Agarwal SR, Malhotra V, Sakhuja P, Sarin SK. Profile of asymptomatic chronic HBV infection in India. The Indian Journal of Medical Research. 2002;**116**:50-57

[16] Satapathy SK, Garg S, Chauhan R, Malhotra V, Sakhuja P, Sharma BC, et al. Profile of chronic hepatitis B virus in children in India: Experience with 116 children. Journal of Gastroenterology and Hepatology. 2006;**21**(7):1170-1176

[17] Nayak NC, Dhar A, Sachdeva R, et al. Association of human hepatocellular carcinoma and cirrhosis

with hepatitis B virus surface and core antigens in the liver. International Journal of Cancer. 1977;**20**:643-654

[18] Tandon BN, Acharya SK, Tandon A. Epidemiology of hepatitis B virus infection in India. Gut. 1996;**38**(suppl 2):S56-S59

[19] Alter HJ, Holland PV, Purcell RH, et al. Posttransfusion hepatitis after exclusion of commercial and hepatitis B antigen-positive donors. Annals of Internal Medicine. 1972;**77**:691-699

[20] Liu C-J, Chen D-S, Chen P-J. Epidemiology of HBV infection in Asian blood donors: Emphasis on occult HBV infection and the role of NAT. Journal of Clinical Virology. 2006;**36**(Suppl. 1): S33-S44

[21] Margolis HS, Alter MJ, Hadler SC. Hepatitis B: Evolving epidemiology and implications for control. Seminars in Liver Disease. 1991;**11**:84-92

[22] Lok AS, McMahon BJ. Chronic hepatitis B. Hepatology. 2007;**45**(2):507-539

[23] Okamoto H, Tsuda F, Sakugawa H, Sastrosoewignjo RI, Imai M, Miyakawa Y, et al. Typing hepatitis B virus by homology in nucleotide sequence: Comparison of surface antigen subtypes. Journal of General Virology. 1988;**69**:2575-2583

[24] Norder H, Hammas B, Lee SD, Bile K, Courouce AM, Mushahwar IK, et al. Genetic relatedness of hepatitis B viral strains of diverse geographical origin and natural variations in the primary structure of the surface antigen. Journal of General Virology. 1998;**74**:1341-1348

[25] Samuel D, Muller R, Alexander G, et al. Liver transplantation in European patients with the hepatitis B surface antigen. The New England Journal of Medicine. 1993;**329**:1842-1847

[26] Kim WR, Poterucha JJ, Kremers WK, et al. Outcome of liver transplantation for hepatitis B in the United States. Liver Transplantation. 2004;**10**:968-974

[27] Perrillo RP, Schiff ER, Davis GL, et al. A randomized, controlled trial of interferon alfa-2b alone and after prednisone withdrawal for the treatment of chronic hepatitis B. The hepatitis interventional therapy group. The New England Journal of Medicine. 1990;**323**:295-301

[28] Lau DT, Everhart J, Kleiner DE, et al. Long-term follow-up of patients with chronic hepatitis B treated with interferon alfa. Gastroenterology. 1997;**113**:1660-1667

[29] Lin S-H, Sheen I-S, Chien R-N, et al. Long-term beneficial effect of interferon therapy in patients with chronic hepatitis B virus infection. Hepatology. 1999;**29**:971-975

[30] Ikeda K, Kobayashi M, Saitoh S, et al. Significance of hepatitis B virus DNA clearance and early prediction of hepatocellular carcinogenesis in patients with cirrhosis undergoing interferon therapy: Long-term follow up of a pilot study. Journal of Gastroenterology and Hepatology. 2005;**20**:95-102

[31] Villeneuve JP, Condreay LD, Willems B, et al. Lamivudine treatment for decompensated cirrhosis resulting from chronic hepatitis B. Hepatology. 2000;**31**:207-210

[32] Fontana RJ, Keeffe EB, Carey W, et al. Effect of lamivudine treatment on survival of 309 north American patients awaiting liver transplantation for chronic hepatitis B. Liver Transplantation. 2002;**8**:433-439

[33] Liaw YF, Sung JJ, Chow WC, et al. Lamivudine for patients with chronic hepatitis B and advanced liver disease. The New England Journal of Medicine. 2004;**351**:1521-1531

[34] Leung NW, Lai CL, Chang TT, et al. Extended lamivudine treatment in patients with chronic hepatitis B enhances hepatitis B e antigen seroconversion rates: Results after 3 years of therapy. Hepatology. 2001;**33**:1527-1532

[35] Carman WF, Zanetti AR, Karayiannis P, et al. Vaccine induced escapemutan of hepatitis B virus. Lancet. 1990;**336**:325-329

[36] Ogata N, Zanetti AR, Yu M, Miller RH, Purcell RH. Infectivity and pathogenicity in chimpanzees of a surface gene mutant of hepatitis B virus that emerged in a vaccinated infant. The Journal of Infectious Diseases. 1997;**175**:511-523

[37] Carman WF, Korula J, Wallace L, MacPhee R, Mimms L, Decker R. Fulminant reactivation of hepatitis B due to envelope protein that escaped detection by monoclonal HBsAg ELISA. Lancet. 1995;**345**:1406-1407

[38] Hsu HY, Chang MH, Ni YH, Lin HH, Wang SM, Chen DS. Surface gen mutants of hepatitis B virus in infants who develop acute or chronic infections despite immunoprophylaxis. Hepatology. 1997;**26**:786-791

[39] Protzer-Knolle U, Naumann U, Bartenschlager R, et al. Hepatitis B virus with antigenically altered hepatitis B surface antigen is selected by high dose hepatitis B immune globulin after liver transplantation. Hepatology. 1998;**27**:254-263

[40] Carman WF, Trautwein C, Van Deursen FJ, et al. Hepatitis B virus envelope variation after transplantation with and without hepatitis B immune globulin prophylaxis. Hepatology. 1996;**24**:489-493

Chapter 2

Hepatitis B Genotyping and Clinical Implication

Damodar Paudel and Sushma Suvedi

Abstract

Hepatitis B is one of the killer diseases and distributed globally. Nepal sandwiched between India and China. China is the country with high prevalence of hepatitis B surface antigen (HBsAg) account 30% of the world's HBsAg carriers, and India which has intermediate HBsAg prevalence accounts 10% of the world's carriers. Nepal has a low prevalence (around 1%) of hepatitis B virus (HBV) infection in general population. A and D genotypes are more prevalent in India, while band C is in China. The survey done in 2012 elaborated the common genes that are A and D and recombinant C/D in Nepal, but the clinical consequences are unclear. The prevalence of hepatitis B is low in Nepal, but it is widely common in intravenous drug users, PLHA, and HCV positive. The implication of HBV genotyping has clinical implication for the treatment. Basically, response of peginterféron, and antiviral drugs (adefovir, lamivudine, telbivudine) in hepatitis B.

Keywords: hepatitis B, genotyping, distribution, clinical implication, management

1. Introduction

About 257 million people were infected chronically with hepatitis B (HBsAg positive), and 887,000 deaths were recorded in 2015 due to hepatitis B virus (HBV)-related liver diseases, mostly from complication with cirrhosis and hepatocellular carcinoma (HCC) indicating an urgent necessity for better ways to prevent such complication of HBV [1]. HBV infection is the tenth leading cause of death and main contributor of HCC, which is ranked the fifth leading cause of cancer in man [2, 3]. HBV can be differentiated from other hepatitis viruses by genotype and subgenotype. HBV sequence differs by >8% form other genotypes and 4–8% nucleotide differences for subgenotypes. Including newly identified genotypes I and J, there are 10 genotypes A–J. Some HBV genotypes are further classified into subgenotypes.

About 30 subgenotypes are available till date. Many studies have reported that different genotypes and subgenotypes show different geographical distribution and are related to disease progression, clinical progression, response to antiviral treatment, and prognosis [4].

As shown in **Figure 1**, genotype A is widespread in sub-Saharan Africa, Northern Europe, and Western Africa; genotypes B and C are common in Asia; genotype C is primarily observed in Southeast Asia and China; genotype D is dominant in Africa, Europe, Mediterranean countries, and India including Nepal. Genotype E is dominant in South Africa. As a minor genotype, genotype G is reported in France, Germany, and the United States; and genotype H is commonly encountered in

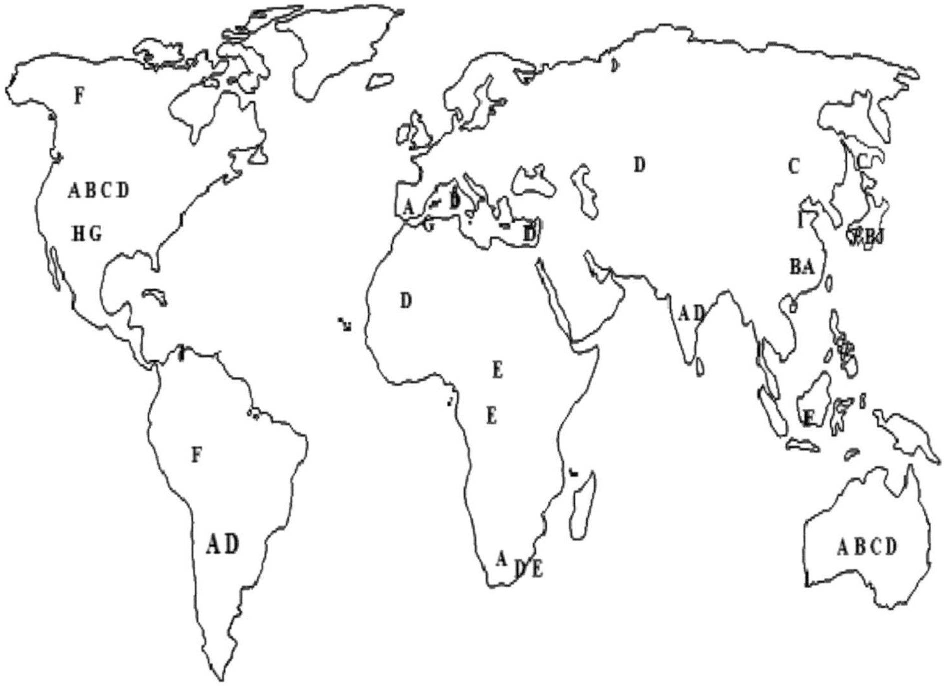

Figure 1.
Global distribution of HBV genotype.

Central and South America and genotype I in Vietnam and Laos. The newest HBV genotype, genotype J, has been identified in the Ryukyu Islands in Japan [5].

However, geographical distribution is still incomplete as data was based on very small numbers of patients and from only few countries.

Nepal is sandwiched between India and China, two countries with high prevalence of hepatitis B surface antigen (HBsAg) positive cases; 30% of the world's HBsAg carriers are in China and 10% in India. Nevertheless, Nepal has a low prevalence (around 1%) of hepatitis B virus (HBV) infection in general population [6]. Hepatitis virus A and D genotypes are dominant in India, while Band C is dominant in China. The prevalence of HBV infection is low in Nepal, but still it is widely common among intravenous drug users, PLHA, and HCV-positive populations. Although our previous study revealed only A, D, and C/D recombinant genotype [8], in the locality of Nepal, all four common genotypes (A, B, C, and D) were reported in the previous study [7].

Phylogenetic tree (**Figure 2**) was obtained from the aligned sequences combining with all human hepatitis B subgenotypes. The Nepal 10 strain was a C/D recombinant genotype, and it is differed from the genotypes A and D or other Nepalese strains. Genotype A1 in Nepal was more similar to that of Bangladesh and the Philippines, while A2 was more similar to the genotype A2 of Japan, Germany, Canada, and Russia. Genotype A1 (Nepal 31, 41, 24, 64, 50, 6, 9, 7, 47 strains) is similar to the A1 genotype of the Philippines, while strain 36, 16, and 18 are more similar to Bangladesh A1 strain. Almost all A1 strains of Nepal showed 88% similarity with Malawi A1 strain. Basically, HBV E genotype of Ghana and Sweden is nearby the genotype D of Nepal. Even some sequences from Germany and Italy are similar to the genotype D of Nepal.

Among genotype D, Nepal 12 and 55 isolates are similar with German D genotype isolates, while Nepal 60 and 57 isolates are more similar with D isolates of Italy and France and Russian isolates of D genotype. These isolates are 93% similar with Nepal 21 f isolates from where the strain Nepal 28 was evolved. Nepal 28 isolates of D genotype is evolved to more similar isolates 22, 32, and 14. Nepal isolates 40, 38

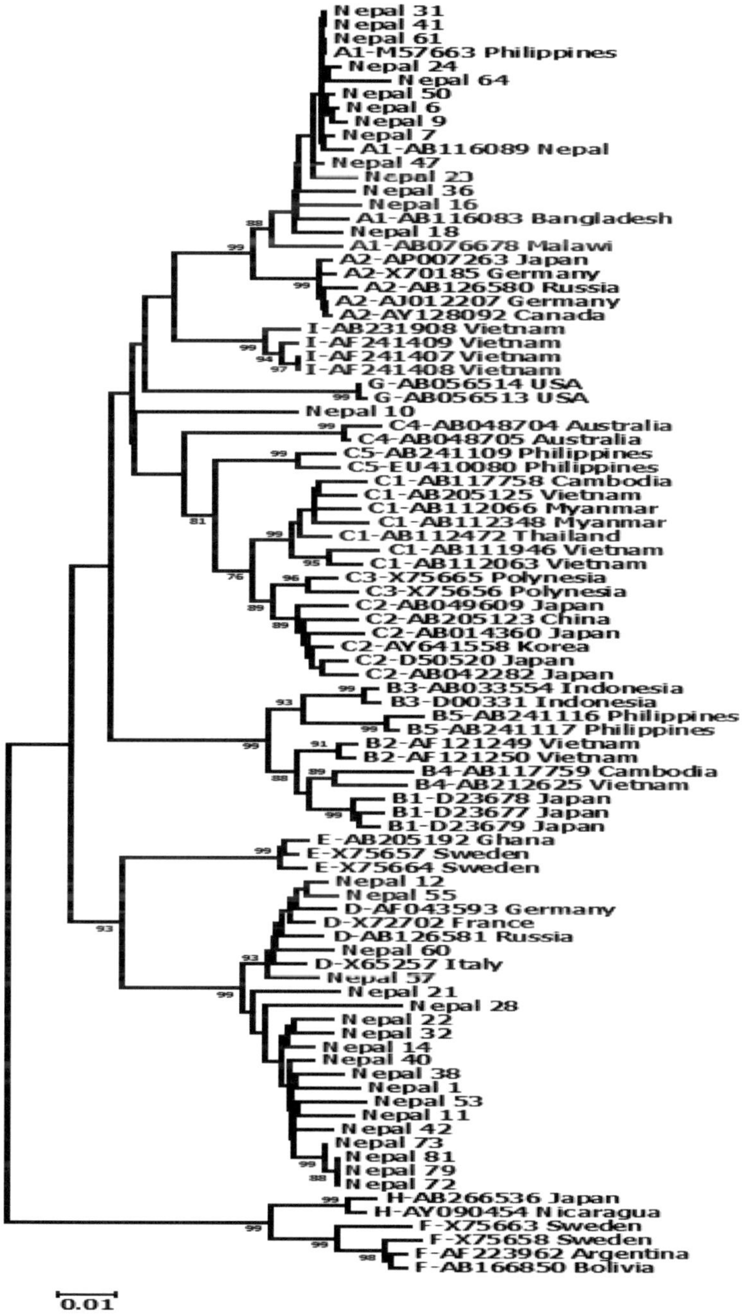

Figure 2.
Phylogenetic tree of Nepal study 2012.

1, 53, 11, 42, and 73 are more similar. Nepal 73 is more similar with 81, 79, and 72, while Nepal 81 and 79 is 88% similar with Nepal 72 isolates [8].

2. Clinical importance of HBV genotypes

As different regions have different serotypes and different clinical spectrum and different molecular epidemiological patterns, different HBV genotypes, but not different rashes, may influence clinical outcome, HBeAg seroconversion rate, mutational patterns in the precore and core promoter regions, and response to interferon therapy [9].

Determination of genotypes: detection of the sequence differences in pre-S or S gene can be done by several methods, e.g., direct sequencing, restriction fragment length polymorphism, line probe assay, genotype-specific PCR, and mass spectrometry.

3. Treatment: noncirrhotic patients

Cirrhosis is defined as distortion of the hepatic architecture and the formation of regenerative nodules. It is generally irreversible in its late stage. It can progress even to hepatocellular carcinoma (HCC). The recommendation for the treatment initiation for cirrhotic patients are available as three different guidelines (EASL 2017, Asia pacific 2015, AASLD 2018) shown in **Table 1** [4, 10, 11].

All patients with compensated cirrhosis HBeAg positive and HBV DNA level >20,000 U/ml with increased ALT twice higher than the normal limit are recommended to be treated by all three regional guidelines. However, AASLD guideline recommends different upper limit of normal (ULN) of ALT in male and female, i.e., 35 and 25, respectively, although EASL and APSL guidelines recommend 40 as ULN of ALT. HBeAg-negative patients with cirrhosis and HBV DNA > 2000 U/ml and the ALT twice higher than normal or the family history of cirrhosis and HCC are also recommended for treatment. EASL recommended to treat patients if fibrosis is present [10–12]. Different guideline recommendations are shown in **Table 1**.

Guideline	HBeAg positive		HBeAg negative		ALT	Family history
	HBV DNA copies/ ml	ALT		HBV DNA copies/ ml		Cirrhosis, HCC
EASL2017	>20,000	Double (40)	30 years	>2000	Double + mod. fibrosis	Cirrhosis, HCC
Asia Pacific 2015	>2000	Double (40)		>2000	Double	
AASLD 2018	>2000	Double (m/F 35/25)	40 years	>2000	Double	Cirrhosis, HCC

Table 1.
Comparison of the recommendation of different guideline treatments of noncirrhotic HBV patients.

4. Treatment: cirrhotic patients

Patients with compensated cirrhosis and HBV DNA level >2000 U/ml are treated per recommendations for immune-active chronic hepatitis B (CHB). All three guidelines recommend to treat patients with decompensated cirrhosis and detectable viral load. In cases of compensated cirrhosis, there is discrepancy among the guidelines. In cases of HBV DNA <2000 copy/ml, AASLD and EASL both recommend to treat irrespective to ALT, whereas APSL recommended to such cases to treat only when ALT is above normal [10–12]. Treatment guideline is shown in **Table 2**.

Guideline	Compensated		Decompensated ALT	
	HBV DNA copies/ml	**ALT**	**HBV DNA copies/ml**	
EASL 2017	If >2000	Irrespective	Detectable	Irrespective
Asia Pacific 2015	>2000, if <2000	↑	Detectable	Irrespective
ASLD 2018	2000	Irrespective	Detectable	Irrespective

Table 2.
Comparison of the recommendation of treatment of different guideline of cirrhotic HBV patients.

5. Clinical characteristics of different genotype are important

Genotype B is a common genotype in Asia. Some characteristics of genotype B are as follows [13–16]:

- Is commonly seen in young age less than 35 years as it is generally transmitted by perinatal or vertical route.
- The conversion from acute to chronic phase is less in this genotype.
- HBeAg seroconversion occurs earlier than genotype C.
- HBsAg seroclearance is faster than genotype C.
- Less patients develop cirrhosis.
- HCC development is less.
- Hepatic decompensation is less.
- HBV DNA is high in number.
- Less chance of getting fulminant hepatitis.

Genotype C is also a common genotype in Southeast Asia and China. Characteristics of genotype care are as follows [13–16]:

- Is commonly seen in young age less than 35 years generally transmitted by perinatal or vertical route.
- The conversion from acute to chronic phase is higher in this genotype.
- HBeAg seroconversion is less percentage and takes time than genotype B.
- HBsAg seroclearance is less than genotype B.
- High chance of getting cirrhosis.
- HCC development is more likely.

- Hepatic decompensation is higher in this genotype.
- HBV DNA is less in copy number.
- Less chance of getting fulminant hepatitis.

Genotype A is distributed worldwide. Characteristics of genotype A are as follows [13–16]:

- It is generally transmitted by horizontal route.
- The conversion from acute to chronic phase is frequent in this genotype.
- HBeAg seroconversion is earlier than genotype D.
- HBsAg seroclearance is also more frequent than genotype D.
- Less patients get cirrhosis.
- HCC development is less.
- Hepatic decompensation is higher.
- HBV DNA is high in copy number.
- Less chance of getting fulminant hepatitis.

Genotype clinical characteristics	B	C	A	D	E–J
Age	Common <35	>35	—	—	
Modes of transmission	Perinatal/vertical	Perinatal/vertical	Horizontal	Horizontal	Horizontal
Chronicity	Lower	Higher	Higher	Lower	—
HBeAg seroconversion	Earlier	Later	Earlier	Later	Earlier
HBeAg seroclearance			Earlier	Later	
HBsAg seroclearance	More	Less	More	Less	_
Cirrhosis	Less active	Active			
HCC	Better	Worse	Better	Worse	Worse in genotype F
HBV DNA level	Higher	Lower	Higher	Lower	_
Hepatic decompensation	Lower	Higher	Higher	Higher	_
Fulminant hepatitis	Less	Less	Less	Higher	

Table 3.
Clinical characteristics of different genotypes of HBV.

Genotype D also has worldwide distribution. Characteristics of genotype D are as follows [13–16].

- Transmitted by horizontal route.
- The conversion from acute to chronic phase is less frequent in this genotype.
- HBeAg seroconversion takes longer time than genotype A.
- HBsAg seroclearance is less than genotype A.
- HCC development is most frequent.
- Hepatic decompensation is higher.
- HBV DNA is low in copy number.
- Higher chance of getting fulminant hepatitis.

Different HBV genotype clinical characteristics are compared in **Table 3**.

6. Antiviral treatment

The goal of therapy

- Decrease ALT—decrease necrotic inflammation in the liver
- Decrease viral load to the undetectable level
- HBeAg seroconversion to generate anti-HBeAg—to minimize the replication of virus
- To reduce HBsAg and seroconversion and anti-HBS
- Prevent development of new esophageal varices

Long-term goal is to reduce the risk of HCC and chronic liver diseases.

Peg-IFN alfa-2a or alfa-2b is recommended before starting peg-IFN therapy to HBeAg-positive patients; good responders should be identified; i.e., low viral load, HBV genotypes A and B, high serum ALT levels (above 2–5 times ULN) and high activity scores on liver biopsy are the predictors for better responding patients.

As the baseline predictor of response for the therapy to HBeAg-negative patient, HBV genotype, HBV DNA, ALT, HBsAg levels, and age are the crucial factors [17].

When to terminate Peg-IFN therapy: if low probability of response for HBeAg positive.

Or

No decline of HBsAg level for HBV genotype A and D at week 12 of treatment.

6.1 HBeAg loss

HBeAg loss with HBV DNA <2000 IU/ml for 6 months after treatment. Genotype D HBeAg-negative patient decreasing <2log decline in HBV DNA at week 12 of peg-IFN therapy [18].

Either entecavir or tenefovir is recommended for HIV

6.2 No response

HBeAg-positive patient with HBsAg level >20,000 IU/ml predicted no response after treatment. HIV positive, TNF + entecavir (lamivudine) + EFV is recommended. Other drugs are recommended as the second-line therapy if the first-line drug treatment is failed (if HBV DNA > log10 IU/ml in 3-month period [19].

6.3 Response to lamivudine

Genotype B has sustain responsiveness to lamivudine followed by genotype C. Genotype A is more resistant than genotype D so that virological responses to the drug are better in genotype D than genotype A. Pediatric patients have good tolerance to lamivudine. The younger the age at diagnosis, the longer consolidation treatment period [20].

6.4 Response to adefovirdipivoxil

Patients infected with genotypes A and D equally respond to 48-week treatment of adefovirdipivoxil, but there could be the adefovir resistance in patients having genotype D.

6.5 Response to entecavir or telbivudine

The relationship of HBV genotypes on drug resistance to entecavir was evaluated in lamivudine-refractory patients. Two-year therapy of telbivudine showed that HBeAg seroconversion, ALT normalization, and HBV negativity were comparable among different genotypes. Entecavir treatment has a chance of HBsAg seroloss in genotypes A and D, and the efficacy is better in Caucasian than in Asian population [20].

6.6 Tenefovir (TDF)

HBsAg loss in genotype A patient followed by genotype D (20 and 10%, respectively) was reported after completion of 144 weeks of treatment of TDF. The therapeutic effect was less in genotypes B and C [20].

Nucleotide analogue	Dose	Adverse	EASL	ASL	APSL
Lamivudine	100 mg/day		Undetectable DNA For 3 years	1–3 years after HBeAg-negative patient	Undetectable DNA For 2 years
Adefovir	10 mg/day				
Entecavir	0.5 mg/day				
Telbivudine	600 mg/day				
Tenofovir	300 mg/day	Bone and renal impairment			
Emcitrabine	200 mg/day				
Tenofovir alafenamide	25 mg/day				

Table 4.
Antiviral treatment doses and period of recommendation by different guidelines.

6.7 Management of incomplete responder

Incomplete responder should be checked for the drug adherence.

Patients who have previous exposure to lamivudine should be considered for entecavir resistance.

EASL recommend to switch to NA or combination therapy if detectable HBV DNA in 12 weeks of therapy. Combination of TDF + ETV has resulted in undetectable DNA even after 4 years, which is better than TDF alone [21]. Most of the study and the guideline do not recommend peg-IFN + nucleot(s)ide therapy, but recommend to use peg-IFN after NA therapy. Antiviral drugs and their continuation recommended by different guideline are illustrated in **Table 4**.

7. Conclusion

HBV genotyping is important for the proper management of chronic HBV patients. Clinical characteristics may be helpful to estimate the genotype and initiate antiviral therapy.

Author details

Damodar Paudel[1]* and Sushma Suvedi[2]

1 Department of Medicine, Internal Medicine Unit, National Academy of Health Science, Nepal Police Hospital, Kathmandu, Nepal

2 Department of Microbiology, Nepalgunj Medical College, Nepalgunj, Nepal

*Address all correspondence to: damodarpaudel@gmail.com

References

[1] WHO, WHO Key facts; 2018

[2] Zamor PJ, deLemos AS, Russo MW. Viral hepatitis and hepatocellular carcinoma: Etiology and management. Journal of Gastrointestinal Oncology. 2017;**8**(2):229-242

[3] Raihan R et al. Hepatocellular carcinoma in Malaysia and its changing trend. Euroasian Journal of Hepato-Gastroenterology. 2018;**8**(1):54-56

[4] Lin CL, Kao JH. Hepatitis B virus genotypes and variants. Cold Spring Harbor Perspectives in Medicine. 2015;**5**(5):a021436

[5] Sunbul M. Hepatitis B virus genotypes: Global distribution and clinical importance. World Journal of Gastroenterology. 2014;**20**(18):5427-5434

[6] Shrestha SM, Shrestha S. Chronic hepatitis B in Nepal: An Asian country with low prevalence of HBV infection. Tropical Gastroenterology. 2012;**33**(2):95-101

[7] Huy TT et al. High prevalence of hepatitis B virus pre-s mutant in countries where it is endemic and its relationship with genotype and chronicity. Journal of Clinical Microbiology. 2003;**41**(12):5449-5455

[8] Paudel D et al. Diversity of hepatitis B genotypes in Nepal and updated phylogenetic tree: A pilot survey in 2012. JNMA; Journal of the Nepal Medical Association. 2014;**52**(196):982-991

[9] Furusyo N et al. Relationship of genotype rather than race to hepatitis B virus pathogenicity: A study of Japanese and Solomon islanders. The American Journal of Tropical Medicine and Hygiene. 2004;**70**(5):571-575

[10] Association, E. EASL 2017 clinical practice guidelines on the management of hepatitis B virus infection. Journal of Hepatology. 2017;**67**(2):370-398

[11] Terrault NA et al. Update on prevention, diagnosis, and treatment of chronic hepatitis B: AASLD 2018 hepatitis B guidance. Hepatology. 2018;**67**(4):1560-1599

[12] Sarin SK et al. Asian-Pacific clinical practice guidelines on the management of hepatitis B: A 2015 update. Hepatology International. 2016;**10**(1):1-98

[13] Kramvis A. The clinical implications of hepatitis B virus genotypes and HBeAg in pediatrics. Reviews in Medical Virology. 2016;**26**(4):285-303

[14] Liaw YF. HBeAg seroconversion as an important end point in the treatment of chronic hepatitis B. Hepatology International. 2009;**3**(3):425-433

[15] Kmet Lunacek N, Poljak M, Maticic M. Distribution of hepatitis B virus genotypes in Europe and clinical implications: A review. Acta Dermatovenerologica Alpina Pannonica et Adriatica. 2018;**27**(3):141-146

[16] Lin CL, Kao JH. The clinical implications of hepatitis B virus genotype: Recent advances. Journal of Gastroenterology and Hepatology. 2011;**26**(Suppl 1):123-130

[17] Liu LZ et al. Improvements in the management of chronic hepatitis B virus infection. Expert Review of Gastroenterology & Hepatology. 2018;**12**(11):1-14

[18] Rijckborst V et al. Early on-treatment prediction of response to peginterferon alfa-2a for HBeAg-negative chronic hepatitis B using HBsAg and HBV DNA levels. Hepatology. 2010;**52**(2):454-461

[19] WHO. Guidelines for the Prevention Care and Treatment of Persons with Chronic Hepatitis B Infection; 2015. Available in https://www.who.int/hiv/pub/hepatitis/hepatitis-b-guidelines/cn/

[20] Man Cho S, Choe BH. Treatment strategies according to genotype for chronic hepatitis B in children. Annals of Translational Medicine. 2016;**4**(18):336

[21] Chan HLY et al. Effects of tenofovir disoproxil fumarate in hepatitis B e antigen-positive patients with normal levels of alanine aminotransferase and high levels of hepatitis B virus DNA. Gastroenterology. 2014;**146**(5):1240-1248

Section 2

Hepatitis C

Chapter 3

Coinfection of Hepatitis B and C in HIV Patients: A Review of the State of the Art

Alexandra Porras-Ramírez and Alejandro Rico-Mendoza

Abstract

Infection with the human immunodeficiency virus (HIV) modifies the course of infection by the virus of hepatitis B (HBV) by several mechanisms: the rate of chronicity, prolonging viremia by HBV, and increase in morbidity related to liver disease. The treatment for both infections should be done in a coordinated manner, to avoid the emergence of resistance in HIV, HBV or both, as well as major alterations in the hepatic enzymes. Monotherapies with lamivudine or emtricitabine select, rapidly, mutant strains of the HBV and HIV. Monotherapy with adefovir has moderate effects in coinfected patients as they already have mutations. If the treatment of HBV can defer until the combination antiretroviral therapy of HIV is necessary, these patients should receive a combination of tenofovir plus lamivudine (or emtricitabine), since this provides a powerful therapy against HBV and establishes a good central axis for antiretroviral therapy. In addition, it would prevent the selection of HBV variant resistance. The influence of HIV in the HCV infection. Increase in load HIV-driven viral hepatitis exacerbates hepatic lesions and influences transmission of the HCV. The risk of sexual transmission increases when HIV is present in the carrier. Coinfection modifies the evolution of fibrosis in patients with HIV, with higher speed in those who have low CD4 counts, so that the onset of cirrhosis occurs before, and the risk of liver decompensation is also more frequent. The consequence of this situation is an increase in liver-related morbidity and mortality.

Keywords: hepatitis B, HIV coinfection, hepatitis C

1. Introduction

The hepatitis B virus is one of the most pathogenic and prevalent in the world. In some places, up to 95% of those infected with HIV have also been infected with hepatitis B, and 10–15% will develop chronic hepatitis B. However, there is a great variation for both infections according to the geographical region and the risk group. In the USA, it is estimated that 100,000 HIV-infected patients suffer from chronic HBV. We do not have data for our country. In patients coinfected with HIV and HBV, HBV is less likely to be eliminated. The infection with primary HBV leads to chronic hepatitis in 2–5% of immunocompetent adults, while patients infected with HIV can become chronic about 5 times more (15–23%). One possible reason is the T-cell defect associated with HIV infection.

IntechOpen

HBV and HIV have several characteristics in common even though HBV is a double-stranded DNA virus. After entering the hepatocyte, viral DNA is integrated into the host genome and the viral RNA is translated by the HBV inverse polymerase in new viral DNA and transcribed to viral proteins. The reverse transcription can be inhibited by nucleic acid (t) transcriptase inhibitors reverse. The integration of the virus into the host's genome in hepatocytes and CD4+ T cells prevents its eradication.

Finally, the mechanisms used to develop resistance are very similar in both viruses. All HIV patients should be screened for HBV and HCV. Screening of HIV-infected patients for HBV must start with the HBsAg application, anti-HBs, and anti-HBc. If a positive HBsAg is found, you must complete the study with HBeAg, anti-HBe, and HBV DNA. On the other hand, for all patients diagnosed with HBV infection, you should have an ELISA for HIV to rule out coinfection.

Like patients monoinfected with HBV with chronic hepatitis B, those coinfected with HIV should be evaluated every 6–12 months for hepatocellular carcinoma, by measuring alpha-fetus protein and performing an ultrasound of the liver. This recommendation is regardless of whether the patient has apparent cirrhosis or not.

The improvement of survival in infected patients by the human immunodeficiency virus (HIV), resulting from the introduction of the therapy powerful antiretroviral ("HAART"), has caused chronic liver infections will become important causes of hospitalization and mortality in patients infected with HIV (HIV+) [1].

Liver diseases and their consequences represent between 30 and 55% of the causes of death in these patients [2]. Frequently, the infection by the viruses of the hepatitis B (HBV) and hepatitis C (HCV) is a cause of chronic liver disease in patients who are HIV+, which can be attributed to the means of transmission and the epidemiological factors among the three viruses [3].

Although the impact of HBV is still not well known in the progression of HIV disease, you have to be very clear about the interference of infection by HIV in the natural history of HBV infection. Coinfected patients have viral loads of HBV that are higher than monoinfected, with a greater risk and a shorter time of evolution to cirrhosis [4].

The presence of HIV modifies the natural history of HCV infection, accelerating the progression of hepatic disease in coinfected people. Of people infected with HCV, between 8 and 24% contract cirrhosis in the first 10–20 years after their HCV infection [5]. The annual incidence of hepatocellular carcinoma of cirrhosis is between 1 and 4% [5].

Works carried out in different countries have shown that the prevalence of HIV/HBV coinfection ranges between 4.8 and 15% [6–8]. In Brazil, according to previous studies in various urban areas, the prevalence of chronic hepatitis B in patients who are HIV+ ranged between 5.3 and 19.2% [9–12]. Studies conducted in several countries reveal that the frequency in the presence of anti-HCV in patients who are HIV+ varies between 0 and 42.5% [6–8].

2. Coinfection with hepatitis B in patients with HIV

Hepatitis B, caused by the hepatitis virus B (HBV), is an important problem of public health and it is the most serious kind of viral hepatitis. It can cause chronic liver disease and carries a high risk of death for cirrhosis and liver cancer. It is estimated that in the world there are 2 billion people infected with HBV and more than 350 million with chronic liver infection [13].

Coinfection of HBV with the human immunodeficiency virus (HIV) is common since they have the same transmission routes.

In Western Europe and in the United States, it has been found that 7–10% of HIV patients have a chronic infection by HBV, with men who have sex with other men being the group with the highest prevalence [14–16]. Patients coinfected with HBV and HIV have an increased risk of liver cirrhosis, terminal liver disease and death by hepatic pathology, especially in patients with low CD4 lymphocyte counts and concomitant use of alcohol [15]. There is a greater risk of hepatocarcinoma and adverse hepatotoxic effects in patients using therapy with highly effective antiretroviral drugs (TARAE) coinfected with hepatitis B [16].

Ninety-five percent of HBV infections in adults who are healthy are self-limiting with an elimination of HBV blood and lasting immunity against the reinfection. Chronic infection happens in less than 5% of patients older than 5 years [14, 17]. Immunosuppressed patients such as patients with HIV, who are in substitution therapy for kidney and diabetics, present a greater risk of chronicity of HBV infection [18–20]. Approximately 15% of patients with chronic infection older than 5 years can evolve into cirrhosis and hepatic cancer, remaining asymptomatic until the appearance of the clinical manifestations of said complications [21]. It is estimated that 20% of HIV-positive patients infected with HBV will develop chronic hepatitis by this agent [18].

The antigens and antibodies associated with the infection of hepatitis B virus are as follows:

A. Surface antigen (HBs Ag): Associated to active infection. Identify patients who are infectious and can be detected from 3 to 5 weeks after the infection. When it remains more than 6 months high, it is related to chronic infection with HBV [22].

B. Antibody against surface antigen (anti-HBs): Its presence indicates in the most of the time, immunity for infection with HBV, natural or acquired, as long as its value is equal or superior to 10 IU/ml (International Units per milliliter) [23].

C. Antibodies against the core of HBV (anti-HBc): The total anti-HBc is considered a marker of the previous infection by HBV. Is composed of two fractions: anticore IgM, appears at the onset of symptoms, up to 30 days after the appearance of HBs Ag, or during the period in which the biochemical tests liver cells are altered in the infection acute and declines between 3 and 12 months after the exhibition; anticore IgG, appears during the acute phase of the disease associated with HBs Ag and persists throughout life of the individual infected with HBV. The presence of anticore IgG can mean: (1) the previous infection with immunity, presence of concomitant antibody to the antigen of serum surface greater than 10 IU/ml. (2) in the previous infection with loss of anti-HBs, these patients have no evidence neither of viral replication nor of antibodies against the surface antigen, because the levels of these antibodies have disappeared over time, but reappear after the application of one or more doses of the vaccine against hepatitis B.

D. HBV infection hidden, are patients with presence of DNA viral serum or liver and absence of HBs Ag and anti-HBs. This situation is not uncommon in patients HIV positive, infection with the virus Hepatitis C and in areas of high prevalence of infection by HBV.

The infection hidden by HBV may be present in 10–45% of HIV-positive patients [24, 25]. Therefore, it is recommended that in all HIV-positive patients the following exams for HBV screening are done: HBs Ag, total anti-HBc or anticore IgG and anti-HBs. If the patient has an isolated positive IgG anticore, it is a must to perform the viral load of HBV DNA. If a patient has anticore IgG positive in isolation and the viral load for HBV is negative, this patient should be vaccinated against hepatitis B and he or she could have an anamnestic or primary response [26, 27].

In patients infected with HIV, atypical serological patterns may appear. More frequent is the isolated presence of anti-HBc (**Table 1**), indicative of hepatitis B cured with loss of antibodies. Exceptionally, it may be hepatitis hidden B, defined by the presence of HBV DNA in liver and serum (viremia will usually be <103 copies/ml and may be intermittent) in patients with negative HBsAg. In the hidden hepatitis B, the markers usually detected are anti-HBc, anti-HBs, and anti-HBe, although these markers can be negative (hepatitis B hid seronegative) 4 in most patients with hidden hepatitis B, the HbeAg is negative4 (**Table 1**).

2.1 The course of concurrent hepatitis B and HIV infection

In HIV-positive patients, chronic hepatitis B has an unfavorable evolution compared with patients infected only with HBV, and the associated mortality risk with hepatopathy is significantly increased. In the MACS study (multicenter AIDS cohort study), coinfected patients had an associated mortality to liver disease 8 times higher than HIV-positive patients HBsAg negative and 15 times greater than patients negative for both infections. Mortality associated with hepatopathy due to hepatitis B has increased, significantly, since the introduction of the highly active antiretroviral therapy (HAART).

In addition to increased mortality, in coinfected patients, HIV accelerates the progression of hepatitis B and increases the risk of cirrhosis significantly. It is important that the clinician is not fooled by the apparent benign course of hepatitis B in HIV patients since this is due to its cellular immunological compromise. Frequently, these patients have only one slight increase in transaminases. However,

Type infection	Anti-HBS	HBsAg	Anti-HBc (IgM)	Anti-HBc (IgG)	HBeAg	Anti-HBe	AND HBV
Acute infection	—	+	+	−/+	+	—	+
Past infection	+/−	—	—	+	—	—	—
Asymptomatic carrier	—	+	—	+	—	−/+	—
Chronic hepatitis B HBeAg+	—	+	—	+	+	—	+
Chronic hepatitis B mutant pre-core	—	+	—	+	—	−/+	+
Occult viral infection positive	+	—	+/−	+	+/−	−/+	+
Occult viral infection negative	—	—	—	—	—	—	+
History of vaccination	+	—	—	—	—	—	—

Table 1.
Serologic markers of HBV and clinical interpretation.

if HBV-DNA is measured, as a marker of viral replication, this is higher in HIV patients than in patients who are immunocompetent.

There is a direct correlation between the degree of immunosuppression and control of HBV replication in the coinfected patients. Patients with AIDS usually show, more frequently, signs of active viral replication. Even in cases with hepatitis B, apparently resolved, progressive deterioration of the immune system can lead to re-activation of an HBV infection. Most studies on the influence of hepatitis B in the evolution of HIV infection have not demonstrated a shortening in survival. The infection with HBV does not lead to a faster reduction of cells CD4+ or increase the frequency of defining diseases of AIDS. However, some interactions do occur. For example, the hepatotoxicity associated with antiretroviral drugs is three times more in patients with chronic HBV hepatitis.

2.2 Prevention

All HIV-infected patients who are serologically negative for HBV should be vaccinated; this should be done despite the fact that the vaccine may be less effective in them. Approximately 30% of patients who are HIV positive are primarily nonresponsive to the vaccine, against 2.5% of immunocompetent individuals. This is especially true for individuals with minor CD4 of 500 cells/mm^3. Therefore, for these patients, a standard vaccination schedule is recommended. If the patient has less than 350 CD4 cells, it is advised to postpone vaccination until after antiretroviral therapy, and patients should be educated in strategies to prevent the progression of liver diseases, such as suppressing consumption of alcohol and tobacco and not using herbal supplement (many of which are hepatotoxic).

Standard vaccination against HBV is less effective in infected patients for HIV. The administration of four doses of 40 μg (months 0, 1, 2, and 6) improves significantly the serological response, and it is the recommended guideline [28].

The consumption of alcohol has an additive effect in terms of progression to fulminant hepatitis, development of aggressive chronic liver disease, and development of hepatocellular carcinoma. Hepatotoxic drugs must be used very carefully and under strict surveillance [29].

2.3 Treatment

HBV-HCV and HBV-HCV-HDV infections are associated with further progression of rapid liver fibrosis [30]. The treatment indications for patients coinfected with HBV-HCV are the 16, same as for each of the infections separately. In patients with multiple infections, there is a predominance of replication (VHD > HCV > HBV) that conditions the detection of viral loads of HBV and HCV lower than in patients without multiple infections [31].

The suppression of HIV replication and immunological improvement secondary to initiation of antiretroviral treatment (ART) is associated with a lower progression of liver disease, even in patients with decompensated cirrhosis [32].

Therefore, ART is a priority in the care of these patients. In those with preserved liver function, any of the drugs recommended in the therapeutic guidelines can be used since the risk of severe hepatotoxicity is low. In child B/C stages, protease inhibitors (PIs) and raltegravir (RAL) are more secure than NEV or EFV [33].

Dolutegravir [34], etravirine [35], and rilpivirine [36] can be used as there is no need to adjust the dose in patients with moderate hepatic insufficiency (child A/B), and in advanced stages, some centers monitor the plasma concentrations of the drugs and adjust their doses. RAL has demonstrated adequate serum levels without the need for dose adjustment and a good tolerance in child [37] stage C patients.

In coinfected patients with HBV/HIV, tenofovir (TDF) suppresses HBV replication in most patients and should be part of the ART, and if there are no contraindications, whenever possible, it will be added as second nucleoside analog (t) gone [33] TC or FTC.

It must be taken into account that simeprevir (SMV) increases TDF levels and, potentially, the risk of nephrotoxicity. In an observational study in patients infected with HIV and coinfected with HBV/HDV, the addition of interferon for 48 weeks to treatment with TDF (n = 4) was associated with a greater decrease in VHD-RNA compared to TDF (n = 13). However, the guideline optimal treatment and response monitoring are not well determined and the clinical relevance of the decrease in VHD-RNA due to IFN is unknown [38].

3. Coinfection with hepatitis C in patients with HIV

The influence of HIV in the HCV infection. Increase in load HIV-driven viral hepatitis exacerbates Hepatic lesions and influences transmission of the HCV. The risk of sexual transmission increases when HIV is present in the carrier. This situation is more evident in the case of homosexual men with multiple sexual contacts without using a preservative [39, 40].

In the case of mother-to-child transmission, the risk of transmission to the fetus in coinfected women for HIV is between 2 and 5 times higher than in mothers monoinfected by HCV and it is between 5 and 25% [41].

Hepatitis C behaves differently in people with HIV, since HIV accelerates the evolution of hepatitis C (even so, many people have lived for many years with a coinfection for HIV and HCV, often without knowing they were coinfected). The risk of significant damage to the liver is greater in people with HIV who have a CD4 count below 200 cells/mm^3. HCV can be treated, regardless of whether the person is or is not infected with HIV. Antiretroviral therapy has reduced notably the number of deaths caused by HIV. Currently, liver disease in the terminal stage produced by coinfection with HCV has become one of the causes of death rates among people living with HIV in certain areas of the United States and Western Europe. In part, this is because HCV infection can go undiagnosed until there has already been serious liver damage.

Coinfection modifies the evolution of fibrosis in patients with HIV, with higher speed in those who have low CD4 counts, so that the onset of cirrhosis occurs before, and the risk of liver decompensation is also more frequent. The consequence of this situation is an increase in liver-related morbidity and mortality [42, 43].

It is confirmed that coinfection by the HIV alters the natural history of HCV, that increases the risk of can become chronic of HCV, accelerates the progression of liver fibrosis associated with VHC [44], increases the risk of decompensation of cirrhosis and decreases survival after the first episode of decompensation. On the contrary, contradictory data have been published about the impact that HCV can have in the natural history of HIV, although does not seem to influence the progression of clinical events defining AIDS or in mortality [45, 46].

The progression of fibrosis is variable and depends on factors related to the causative agent and factors related to the host. Among these factors, consumption of alcohol, age at acquisition of infection, race, viral coinfections like the concomitant infection with HIV, time of infection, body mass index, and various genetic factors have been described [22]. Among these, the studies in animals have identified some determinant genetic progression of fibrosis; as well in humans, we have tried to identify polymorphism genetics to predict the degree of progression in hepatitis C and in steatosis of a nonalcoholic liver [47]. Therefore, there are a number of factors that you can modify to prevent the progression of liver fibrosis, including alcohol intake and other toxins, the normalization of the index of body mass, and the prevention of infections for other hepatotropic viruses.

Hepatitis C does not make HIV worse, but it can complicate your treatment, since many drugs to treat HIV metabolize in the liver. Coinfected people have more risk of developing hepatotoxicity associated with the antiretroviral treatment than those who only have HIV. In any case, the benefits of HIV treatment outweigh the risk of hepatic toxicity [48].

HCV screening tests are recommended to all people with HIV. Even if you have already been diagnosed with coinfection with HIV and HCV, it is important to know how HCV is diagnosed and controlled. Unlike HIV, a positive result in the HCV antibody test does not always mean that the person has a chronic infection [48].

HCV screening tests consist of two stages. As usual, first, a test for the detection of antibodies against HCV is carried out. If the result is positive, this means that you have been infected by hepatitis C before and possibly still have. People who eliminated hepatitis C spontaneously without treatment still have the antibodies for many years afterwards. On the other hand, in some cases, the results of the antibodies screening tests are negative even when the person has a chronic infection of hepatitis C. This can happen if [48]:

- the CD4 cell count is low (usually less than 200), since it is possible that the immune system is not producing antibodies; or

- the screening test is performed very shortly after having been infected, since antibodies take between 6 and 24 weeks to develop.

An HCV RNA (viral load) screening test is needed to confirm the existence of a chronic infection (by HCV). The test of viral load searches for genetic material of HCV in the same way that HIV viral load test is used to detect this virus. If the quantity of HCV RNA in the bloodstream is detectable, it means that is currently infected with HCV. If on the other hand it is undetectable, a second test must be performed after 6 months. Yes, if the viral load is not detected in two successive tests, it means that the person has eliminated HCV from the body (**Table 2**) [48].

3.1 Prophylaxis

Serology should be performed against HAV and HBV to all adult patients infected with HIV, and even more so if infection coexists with HCV in order to vaccinate, if appropriate, after having carried out the immunological study. In patients with susceptible HIV, the vaccine against hepatitis A will be administered in a two-dose

Diagnosis	Previous infection and eliminated by hepatitis C virus	Acute infection by hepatitis C virus	Chronic infection by hepatitis C virus
Detection of antibodies	Positive	Negative, is positive 6–24 weeks	Positive
Detection of viral load (HCV RNA)	Undetectable in two tests performed, at least 6 months apart	Detectable in 1 or 2 weeks, usually at very high levels	Detectable
ALT test (alanine aminotransferase)	It can be normal, fluctuate, or show a high level of persistent way	It can be between 7 and 10 times higher than the normal level	It can be normal from persistent way, fluctuate, or show a high level of persistent way

Table 2.
Diagnosis of HCV and clinical interpretation.

schedule separated by 6 months at patients presenting figures > 200 CD4/ml. With those who are in a degree of older immunosuppression, you should wait until your CD4 numbers increase above the 200 cells/ml. There are no recommendations about when to perform the revaccination.

The standard vaccination guideline against HBV is three doses intramuscularly in the deltoids at 0, 1, and 6 months, which produce immunity greater than 90%. The answers are worse particularly among those with lower CD4 [49]. It has been postulated that doubling the standard doses or administering another dose could produce more adequate protection titles [50]. Patients with CD4 < 200 will proceed to vaccination when the figure has increased.

Immunization with the vaccine is lost with time, so controls must be carried out later to check the protection. Controls will be carried out between 4 and 12 weeks after finishing the vaccination, and more lately once a year.

3.2 Treatment for genotype 1 of hepatitis C

The evidence supports that the beginning of the antiretroviral therapy and, therefore, controlling early replication of HIV and maintaining a good immunological situation are the first measures to adopt in the coinfected patients. Existing data indicate that antiretroviral treatment can slow down the progression of chronic HCV liver disease in the coinfected patient, even in the carriers of liver disease, increasing their survival [51, 52].

Studies based on liver biopsies have demonstrated a relationship between the management of antiretroviral treatment, immunological improvement, and the presence of lower grades of hepatic fibrosis [53, 54].

3.2.1 Boceprevir or telaprevir + PR

In patients coinfected with HIV and HCV genotype 1 and without previous treatment for HCV SVR after treatment with Boceprevir (BOC) or telaprevir (TVR) was higher (63–74%) than in those treated with PR (29–45%) [55, 56].

Efficacy and side effects with both triple patterns were similar to those observed in monoinfected patients. The dose of RBV was 800 mg/d in almost all patients. Although significant pharmacokinetic interactions have been described, the co-administration of lopinavir/r, atazanavir/r, and darunavir/r, allowed in the study with PR/BOC, did not affect efficacy [55].

The results of the Unite 115 study support the dosage of TVR every 12 h in coinfected patients and ART based on IP/r or raltegravir, as well as the possibility of shortening the duration to 24 weeks (T12 + PR24) in patients without cirrhosis with HCV-RNA undetectable in S4 and S12.

In pretreated coinfected patients, the results of observational studies are similar to those obtained in clinical trials with monoinfected patients. The efficacy of these guidelines is insufficient in cirrhotic patients or patients with previous response to partial or null P/R. Due to its limited efficacy and high toxicity, treatment with BOC and TVR should be considered for exceptional use, in patients with genotype 1, without treatment or with recurrence prior to PR, when the guidelines considered preferred are not available or alternatives:

1. P/R + TVR × 12 s + P/R× 36 s. (AI). If undetectable viral load in s4 and s12, in absence of cirrhosis: P/R× 24 s (BI)

2. P/R× 4 s (lead-in) + P/R + BOC× 44 s (BI)

3.2.2 Sofosbuvir (SOF) + PR

In the study NEUTRINO [57], 291 patients infected with HCV, genotype 1, without prior treatment, received treatment with SOF + PegIFN alpha-2a + RBV (1000–1200 mg/d) during 12 weeks. Overall, 89% of patients with genotype 1 reached RVS12: subtype 1a, 92% (207/225); subtype 1b, 82% (54/66). The RVS12s was lower in cirrhotic patients (80%) than in noncirrhotic patients (92%).

In a multinational observational study (HCV-TARGET) [58], two thousand and sixty-three patients were analyzed treated with guidelines based on SOF, in combination with PR or with SMV±RBV (in patients with genotype 1) or in combination with RBV (in patients with genotypes 2 or 3); 48% were cirrhotic, 52% pretreated, and 18% with failure prior to triple treatment with PR + IP. Overall, 5.7% of patients had serious side effects (12 patients died and 9 of them were cirrhotic).

In this study, 85% (140/164) of patients with genotype 1 (45% pretreated; 27% pretreated with PR + IP) treated for 12 weeks with SOF + PR obtained an RVS4. SVR4 was higher in noncirrhotic patients (90%) than in cirrhotic patients (70%).

In the observational study TRIO [59] (n = 295, with genotype 1), the SVR 12 s global in patients without previous treatment (analysis by an intention of treatment) was 77%, without differences between cirrhotic patients (81%; 112/138) or not (81%, 25/31). In patients with previous failure (RN: 36%), RVS12 was 72% (90/125): 76% in noncirrhotic patients (n = 39) and 62% in cirrhotic patients (n = 85). Based on the previous regimen, RVS12 was 73% in patients with failure prior to IP + PR (n = 40) and 67% in patients with failure prior to PR (n = 36). Two percent of the patients abandoned the treatment because of side effects.

3.2.3 Simeprevir (SMV) + PR

In the QUEST-1 [60] clinical trials and QUEST-2 [61], the efficacy and safety of SMV (150 mg/d) + PR versus placebo + PR for 24 or 48 weeks (according to criteria of TGR) in patients monoinfected by HCV genotype 1 without previous treatment, the RVS24s overall was 80–81% for SMV + PR and 50% for PBO + P/R. SVR in patients infected with HCV subtype 1a with and without the Q80K polymorphism in the protease was 58% and 84%, respectively. The SVR obtained by patients with subtype 1b was 85% (228/267) globally and 90% (172/192) in the subgroup of European patients included in both studies. Depending on the degree of basal fibrosis, they reached SVR 84% (317/378) of the patients with fibrosis F0-F2, 73% (60/82) with F3, and 60% of the patients with cirrhosis.

A remarkable aspect is the predictive value of the response obtained with this guideline in week 4 of treatment. Of the 521 patients who started treatment with SMV in the QUEST studies, 78% (404/521) showed an RVR, and of them, 90% (362/404) reached RVS12.

In the study TMC435-C212 [62], 106 patients coinfected with HIV/HCV were analyzed treated with SMV/PR, with overall RVS12s of 74%; without previous treatment (n = 53): 79%; previous relapse (n = 15): 87%; RP (n = 10): 70%; RN (n = 28): 57%. Eighty-nine percent of patients without previous treatment or with recurrence, he obtained an RVR and of this 89%, he reached RVS12s. Treatment with SMV + PR was generally well tolerated, with a tolerability profile and safety similar to those shown in monoinfected patients.

In the PROMISE [63] study, patients monoinfected by HCV with recurrence were randomized previously after P/R, to treatment with SMV (n = 260) versus placebo (n = 133) during 12 weeks, with P/R (24–48 weeks). The RVS12s was 86% (128/149) in patients with subtype 1b and 70% (78/111) in those with subtype 1a (78% and 47% in patients without and with the Q80K polymorphism, respectively). Ninety-three percent obtained an RVRe and shortened the total duration of treatment at 24 weeks.

In the ATTAIN study [64], the noninferiority of SMV versus TVR was demonstrated, in combination with PR, in infected or monoinfected patients with partial or no response to RP. Based on the previous response, the SVR obtained was: patients with previous RP, 70% (163/234) with SMV versus 68.5% (163/238) with TVR; patients with previous RN, 44% (63/145) with SMV versus 47% (67/146) with TVR10. The risk of anemia was 3 times smaller in those treated with SMV, being also of a milder character than that that occurred in the TVR group.

3.3 Treatment for genotypes 2 and 3 of hepatitis C

3.3.1 PEGIFN + RBV

In patients coinfected with HIV/HCV genotypes 2/3, the probability of reaching an SVR with pegIFN-alpha-2a (180 μg/week) or alpha-2b (1.5 μg g/kg/week) and adjusted RBV weight (800–1200 mg/d) for 48 weeks is 62–71% [65, 66].

Patients without cirrhosis who achieve an RVR can be treated for 24 weeks without reduction of response rates [67, 68]. In patients with genotype 2 or 3, without previous treatment, due to the lower efficacy and toxicity associated with prolonged administration, treatment with PR should be considered for exceptional use, when the guidelines considered are not available preferred or alternative:

PR × 48 s (BI). In patients with RVR, PR × 24 s, in the absence of cirrhosis (BII).

3.3.2 SOF + RBV

In four clinical studies, phase III, with monoinfected patients with genotype 2, treated with SOF/RBV for 12 weeks, the SVR ranged between 86 and 97% [57, 60, 69]. Also, in the PHOTON 1 [70] studio in patients without prior treatment coinfected with genotype 2, the treatment with SOF/RBV for 12 weeks showed an RVS12 of 88% (23/26); in patients pretreated, the SVR after 24 weeks of treatment was 92%.

Although the data are inconclusive, pretreated cirrhotic patients could benefit from a treatment of more than 12 weeks. In the FUSION study, in patients, the SVR was pretreated 60% (6/10) in cirrhotic patients treated for 12 weeks and 78% (7/9) in those treated for 16 weeks [60].

3.3.3 SOF + DCV

In study AI444-040 89% (16/18) of the monoinfected with genotype 3, without treatment previous, non-cirrhotic, treated with SOF (400 mg/d) + DCV (60 mg/d) ± RBV during 24 weeks, he obtained an SVR, with no apparent impact of the inclusion or not of RBV in the effectiveness [70].

In the ALLY 3 study, 152 patients infected with HCV genotype 3 were treated with SOF 400 mg/d + DCV 60 mg/d for 12 weeks. Overall, they obtained an RVS12 on 90% (91/101) of patients without previous treatment: cirrhotic: 58% (11/19); without cirrhosis: 97% (73/75). Eighty-six percent (44/51) of the pretreated reached RVS12: cirrhotic, 69% (9/13); noncirrhotic, 94% (32/34) [71].

3.4 Treatment for genotype 4 of hepatitis C

3.4.1 PEGIFN ALFA + RBV

Overall, the probability of SVR of patients coinfected with genotype 4 to standard treatment with PR is less than 30% (**Table 1**) 1–5, although it is higher in patients with IL28B CC [32].

3.4.2 SOF + PR

We do not have information with the new direct antivirals in patients coinfected. In patients monoinfected with HCV, the analysis of patients with genotype 4 included in the Neutrino7 study showed an RVS12 of 96% (27/28) after 12 weeks of treatment with SOF + PR (1000–1200 mg/d).

3.4.3 SOF + RBV

In another study [72] in patients of Egyptian descent, the efficacy of SOF 400 mg/day + RBV (1000–1200 mg/day) for 24 weeks was greater than the 12-week schedule, in patients without previous treatment, 100% (14/14) versus 79% (11/14), as in pretreated, 93% (14/15) versus 59% (10/17).

In the Photon 2 [73] study, 84% (26/31) of patients coinfected with genotype 4, without pretreatment, treated with SOF + RBV for 24 weeks obtained an SVR: noncirrhotic 83% (19/23); cirrhotic 88% (7/8).

3.4.4 Interactions between medications

Boceprevir is a potent CYP3A4/5 cytochrome inhibitor. Exposure to medicinal products metabolized by CYP3A4/5 may increase when administered with BOC, which could increase or prolong its therapeutic effects and adverse reactions. BOC is partially metabolized by CYP3A4/5. The joint administration of BOC with drugs that induce or inhibit activity of CYP3A4/5 could increase or decrease exposure to Boceprevir [74]. Boceprevir is contraindicated when co-administered with drugs whose elimination is highly dependent on CYP3A4/5 and in which the elevation of plasma concentrations is associated with serious adverse events or they pose a vital risk. This is the case of midazolam, triazolam, bepridil, pimozide, lumefantrine, halofantrine, lovastatin, quetiapine, alfuzosin, silodosin, and derivatives ergotamines [74].

Telaprevir is partially metabolized by CYP3A and is a substrate of the glycoprotein-P (gp-P). Co-administration of Telaprevir with CYP3A-inducing drugs and/or gp-P can reduce plasma concentrations of TVR. On the contrary, its co-administration with CYP3A inhibitor drugs and/or gp-P may increase plasma concentrations of Telaprevir. On the other hand, Telaprevir is an inhibitor potent of CYP3A4 and gp-P. This inhibition is time dependent and can be intensified during the first 2 weeks of treatment. At the end of the treatment, it may be necessary that approximately 1 week elapses for the inhibitory effect of Telaprevir to disappear. Telaprevir administration can increase the systemic exposure to drugs that are substrates of CYP3A or of gp-P, which may lead to an increase or prolongation of its effects and risk of adverse reactions [75].

Simeprevir is metabolized by CYP3A4. Therefore, the co-administration of Simeprevir with inhibitors of CYP3A4 can increase their plasma concentrations, and in contrast, co-administration of Simeprevir with CYP3A-inducing drugs can reduce plasma concentrations of Simeprevir [76]. Its use is not recommended combined with other nonanalog reverse transcriptase inhibitor nucleosides [76, 77]. The use of SMV with HIV protease inhibitors enhanced or not with ritonavir [77].

Sofosbuvir is a substrate of the gp-P. Therefore, drugs or products that are powerful inducers of gp-P (rifampicin, S Juan's herb, carbamazepine, and phenytoin) can reduce plasma concentrations of SOF and reduce its therapeutic effect. The interactions of Sofosbuvir with antiretroviral drugs have been investigated in a phase 1 clinical trial conducted in healthy volunteers [78]. Sofosbuvir modified the pharmacokinetics of antiretrovirals evaluated within the limits of the prespecified equivalency interval [79].

The interaction between Sofosbuvir and recent integrase inhibitors has not been evaluated; however, the existence of interactions has not foreseen significant differences between Sofosbuvir and these drugs [78].

Daclatasvir is a substrate of CYP3A4 and gp-P. Inducers of CYP3A4 and of gp-P can reduce plasma levels and the therapeutic effect of DCV. The co-administration with potent inducers of CYP3A4 and gp-P is contraindicated, while it is recommended to adjust your dose when used with moderate inductors. Inhibitors of CYP3A4 can increase plasma levels of DCV, so it is recommended to adjust their dose [80]. Daclatasvir has a scarce influence on cytochrome CYP3A4, so that its administration does not affect relevant to the metabolism of antiretroviral drugs and, therefore, adjustment of these is not required.

The administration of efavirenz induces the metabolism of daclatasvir reducing your AUC by approximately 50%. Therefore, it is necessary to increase the dose of daclatasvir at 90 mg/day in case of concomitant use with efavirenz. On the contrary, atazanavir/ritonavir increases the daclatasvir by 2.1 times and, consequently, it is required to reduce the dose of daclatasvir at 30 mg. Daclatasvir/ritonavir increases to a lesser extent the AUC of daclatasvir, by 40%, so it would not require dose adjustment of daclatasvir [81]. The dosage of daclatasvir is the same for ATV/r or DRV/r that for atazanavir or darunavir powered with cobicistat (COBI); that is, the doses of daclatasvir are 30 mg/day co-administered with atazanavir/cobicistat and 60 mg/day with daclatasvir/cobicistat [81]. No relevant interactions between tenofovir disoproxil fumarate and daclatasvir have been observed [80].

4. Summary of hepatitis C treatment according to the genotype

In **Table 3**, you can see the summary of hepatitis C treatment according to the genotype.

5. Conclusions

The influence of HIV in the HCV infection. Increase in load HIV-driven viral hepatitis exacerbates hepatic lesions and influences transmission of the HCV. The risk of sexual transmission increases when HIV is present in the carrier. This situation is more evident in the case of homosexual men with multiple sexual contacts without using a preservative [39, 40].

In the case of mother-to-child transmission, the risk of transmission to the fetus in coinfected women for HIV is between 2 and 5 times higher than in mothers monoinfected by HCV and it is between 5 and 25% [41].

Coinfection modifies the evolution of fibrosis in patients with HIV, with higher speed in those who have low CD4 counts, so that the onset of cirrhosis occurs before, and the risk of liver decompensation is also more frequent. The consequence of this situation is an increase in liver-related morbidity and mortality [42, 43].

Genotype hepatitis C virus	Treatment	Indications	Contraindications	Doses
Genotype 1 (1a or 1b) and 4, 5 or 6	Ledipasvir + sofosbuvir	Patient with chronic hepatitis C genotype 1 (1a and 1b), 4, 5, or 6, with the following characteristics: • No cirrhosis or compensated cirrhosis (child A) or decompensated (child B and C) and • Without prior treatment or with previous treatment with peg-IFN and RBV or with previous treatment with inhibitors of first-generation proteases (Telaprevir or Boceprevir) • Patient with HIV coinfection and the same characteristics considered, taking into account the drug interactions and dose adjustments according to the antiretroviral	• Patient with genotype 2 or 3 • Patient with chronic renal failure with creatinine clearance <30 ml/min	90 mg LDV + 400 mg SOF
Genotype 1 (1a or 1b) and 2 or 3	Daclatasvir + sofosbuvir	• Patient with chronic hepatitis C genotype 1 (1a and 1b), 2, and 3, with the following characteristics: • No cirrhosis or compensated cirrhosis (child A) or decompensated (child B and C) and without prior treatment or with previous treatment with peg-IFN and RBV or with previous treatment with inhibitors of first-generation proteases (Telaprevir or Boceprevir) • Patient with HIV coinfection and the same mentioned characteristics, taking into account the drug interactions and dose adjustments according to the antiretroviral	Patient with chronic renal failure with creatinine clearance <30 ml/min	60 mg DCV + 400 mg SOF

Genotype hepatitis C virus	Treatment	Indications	Contraindications	Doses
Genotype 1 (1a or 1b)	Panitaprivir+ ombitasvir + ritonavir + dasabuvir	Patient with chronic hepatitis C genotype 1 (1a or 1b) with the following characteristics: • No cirrhosis or compensated cirrhosis (child A) and • Without prior treatment or with previous treatment with peg-IFN and RBV • Patient with HIV coinfection and the same mentioned characteristics, taking into account the drug interactions and dose adjustments according to the antiretroviral. Patient with the same characteristics mentioned, and with advanced chronic renal failure (clearance of creatinine <30 mL/min-80 mL/min) or in therapy renal replacement	• Patient with genotype 2, 3, 5, or 6 Patient with decompensated cirrhosis (child B or C)	150 mg PTV + 25 mg OBV + 100 mg r + 500 mg dasabuvir
Genotype 1b	Daclatasvir + asunaprevir	• Patients with chronic hepatitis C genotype 1b with the following characteristics: • No cirrhosis or compensated cirrhosis (child A) and without prior treatment or with previous treatment with peg-IFN and RBV	• Patient with genotype 1a, 2, 3, 4, 5, or 6 • Patient with polymorphism of the N5SA • Patients previously treated with inhibitors of first-generation proteases (Telaprevir or Boceprevir)	60 mg DVC + 100 mg asunaprevir

DOI: http://dx.doi.org/10.5772/intechopen.83704

Genotype hepatitis C virus	Treatment	Indications	Contraindications	Doses
Genotype 1	Simeprevir + Ribavarina	Patient with chronic hepatitis C genotype 1, with following characteristics: • No cirrhosis or compensated cirrhosis (child A) and • Without previous treatment or with previous treatment with peg-IFN and RBV	Patient with chronic renal failure with creatinine clearance <30 ml/min. Patient with all the following characteristics: • Genotype 1a • Cirrhosis • - Q80K polymorphism	150 mg SMV + 400 mg SOF
Genotype 2	Sofosbuvir + Ribavarina	Patient with chronic hepatitis C genotype 2, with the following characteristics: • No cirrhosis or compensated cirrhosis (child A) and • Without prior treatment or with previous treatment with peg-IFN and RBV	• Patient with chronic renal failure with creatinine clearance <30 ml/min • Patient with anemia • Caution should be exercised with the use of RBV in patients of childbearing age, because if it is teratogenic, you must wait at least 6 months after its use to consider pregnancy	400 mg SOF + 1000 mg RBV (if the patient's weight is less than 75 kg) or 1200 mg of RBV. If the weight of the patient is greater than or equal to 75 kg)
Genotype 3	Sofosbuvir + Ribavarina + Peg-IFN	Patient with chronic hepatitis C genotype 3, with the following characteristics: • No cirrhosis or compensated cirrhosis (child A) and • Without prior treatment or with previous treatment with peg-IFN and RBV or with previous treatment with SOF + RBV	• Patient with chronic renal failure with creatinine clearance <30 ml/min • Patient with previous intolerance or effects secondary to pegylated interferon • Patient with anemia. Caution should be exercised with the use of RBV in patients of childbearing age, because if it is teratogenic, you must wait at least 6 months after its use to consider pregnancy	401 mg SOF + 1000 mg RBV + 180 mcg peg-IFN (if the patient's weight is less than 75 kg) or 1200 mg of RBV (If the weight of the patient is greater than or equal to 75 kg)

Genotype hepatitis C virus	Treatment	Indications	Contraindications	Doses
Genotype 4	Sofosbuvir + Ribavarina	Patient with chronic hepatitis C genotype 4, with the following characteristics: • No cirrhosis or compensated cirrhosis (child A) and • Without prior treatment or with previous treatment with peg-IFN and RBV	• Patient with chronic renal failure with creatinine clearance <30 ml/min • Patient with anemia • Caution should be exercised with the use of RBV in patients of childbearing age, because if it is teratogenic, you must wait at least 6 months after its use to consider pregnancy	400 mg SOF + 1000 mg RBV (if the patient's weight is less than 75 kg) or 1200 mg of RBV (If the weight of the patient is greater than or equal to 75 kg)

Table 3.
Treatment of hepatitis C according to genotype.

Acknowledgements

The authors acknowledge Universidad El Bosque for supporting the writing process of this chapter.

Alexandra Porras-Ramírez y Alejandro Rico-Mendoza express:

- Substantially contribute to the conception or design of the work; or the acquisition, analysis, or interpretation of data for the work
- Participate in drafting or revising the work
- Approve the final version of the work to be published.

Conflict of interest

The authors express no conflicts of interest.

Acronyms and abbreviations

BCV	boceprevir
BEC	beclabuvir
DCV	daclatasvir
FVD	faldaprevir
IFN	interferon
Peg-IFN/RBV	peginterferon or pegylated IFN + ribavirina
LDV	ledipasvir
OBV	ombitasvir
Peg-IFN	peginterferon
PTV	paritaprevir
r	ritonavir
RBV	ribavirina
SMV	simeprevir
SOF	sofosbuvir
TDF	tenofovir
TLV	telaprevir

Author details

Alexandra Porras-Ramírez* and Alejandro Rico-Mendoza
Grupo de Medicina Comunitaria y Salud Colectiva, Universidad El Bosque, Bogotá, Colombia

*Address all correspondence to: porras.alexandra@gmail.com

References

[1] Puoti M, A. M. Hepatitis B vírus co-infection in human immunodeficiency virus-infected subjects. AIDS Reviews. 2002;**4**:27-35

[2] Andersson K, C. R. Hepatitis C virus in HIV-infected patient. Clinics in Liver Disease. 2006;**10**:303-320

[3] Kim AY, C. R. Human immuno-deficiency virus and hepatitis B and C coinfection: Pathogenic interactions, natural history and therapy. AIDS Clinical Review. 2000-2001:263-306

[4] Benhamou Y, B.M. Liver fibrosis progression in human immunodeficiency virus and hepatitis C virus coinfected patients. Hepatology. 1999:1054-1058

[5] El-Serag HB, M A, C K. Trends in survival of patients with hepatocellular carcinoma between 1977 and 1996 in the United States. Hepatology. 2001;**625-628**:62-65

[6] D L, Petoumenos K, D G. HIV/HBV and HIV/HCV coinfection and outcomes following highly active antiretroviral therapy. HIV Medicine. 2003:241-249

[7] Ockenga J, Tillmann HL, Trautwein C, Stoll M. Hepatitis B and C in HIV-infected patients. Journal of Hepatology. 1997:18-24

[8] Smikle MF, H. O-H. A serosurvey of hepatitis B virus, hepatitis C virus, human T lymphotropic virus type-1 and syphilis in HIV-1-infected patients in Jamaica. The West Indian Medical Journal. 2003:14-17

[9] Mendes-Correa MCJ, B. A. Prevalence of Hepatitis B and C in the será of patients with HIV infection in São Paulo, Brazil. Revista do Instituto de Medicina Tropical de São Paulo. 2000:81-85

[10] Nuñez M, S V. Management of patients co-infected with hepatitis B vírus and HIV. The Lancet Infectious Diseases. 2005:374-382

[11] MG S, Passos ADC, M A. Co-infecção HIV e vírus da hepatite B: prevalência e fatores de risco. Revista da Sociedade Brasileira de Medicina Tropical. 2004;**37**:391-395

[12] Morimoto HK, A. C-A. Soroprevalência de infecção por hepatite B, hepatite C e HTLV em população infectada pelo HIV/AIDS de Londrina e região. Goiania: Anais do XIII Congresso Brasileiro de Infectologia; 2003

[13] Organización Mundial de la Salud. Hepatitis B. 2008. Obtenido de: http://www.who.int/mediacentre/factsheets/fs204/es/print.html

[14] Edmunds WJ, M. G. The influence of age on the development of the hepatitis B carrier state. Proceedings of the Biological Sciences. 1993;**253**(1337):197-201

[15] Thio CL, S. E. HIV-1, hepatitis B virus, and risk of liver-related mortality in the multicenter cohort study (MACS). Lancet. 2002:1921-1926

[16] Weber R, Sa C-M-S. Liver-related deaths in persons infected with the human immunodeficiency virus: The D:A:D study. Archives of Internal Medicine. 2006:1632-1641

[17] McMahon BJ, A. W. Acute hepatitis B virus infection: Relation of age to the clinical expression of disease and subsequent development of the carrier state. The Journal of Infectious Diseases. 1985:599-603

[18] Hadler SC, J. F. Outcome of hepatitis B virus infection in homosexual men and its relation to prior human immunodeficiency virus infection.

The Journal of Infectious Diseases. 1991;**163**(3):454-459

[19] Hyams. Risks of chronicity following acute hepatitis B virus infection: A review. Clinical Infectious Diseases. 1995;**20**(4):992-1000

[20] Polish LB, S. C. Nosocomial transmission of hepatitis B virus associated with the use of a spring-loaded finger-stick device. The New England Journal of Medicine. 1992:721-725

[21] Goldstein ST, Z. F. A mathematical model to estimate global hepatitis B disease burden and vaccination impact. International Journal of Epidemiology. 2005:1329-1339

[22] Hoofnagle JH, D. B. Serologic diagnosis of acute and chronic viral hepatitis. Seminars in Liver Disease. 1991:73-83

[23] Alward WL, M. B. The long-term serological course of asymptomatic hepatitis B virus carriers and the development of primary hepatocellular carcinoma. Journal of Infectious Diseases. 1985;**151**(4):604-609

[24] Hofer M, H J-J. Frequent chronic hepatitis B virus infection in HIV-infected patients positive for antibody to hepatitis B core antigen only. Swiss HIV Cohort Study. European Journal of Clinical Microbiology & Infectious Diseases. 1998:6-13

[25] Piroth L, B C. The evolution of hepatitis B virus serological patterns and the clinical relevance of isolated antibodies to hepatitis B core antigen in HIV infected patients. Journal of Hepatology. 2002;**36**(5):681-686

[26] Koziel MJ, P. M. Viral hepatitis in HIV infection. The New England Journal of Medicine. 2007:1445-1454

[27] Santos EA, Y. C. Frequent occult hepatitis B virus infection in patients infected with human immunodeficiency virus type 1. European Journal of Clinical Microbiology & Infectious Diseases. 2003:92-98

[28] Launay O, v d. ANRS HB03 VIHVAC BTrial. Safety and immunogenicity of 4 intramuscular double doses and 4 intradermal low doses vs standardhepatitis B vaccine regimen in adults with HIV-1: Randomized controlled trial. JAMA. 2011:1432-1440

[29] Russell M, P M. The impact of lifetime alcohol use on hepatitis C treatment outcomes in privately insured members of an integrated health care plan. Hepatology. 2012:432-440

[30] Lacombe K, R. J. HIV and viral hepatitis coinfections: Advances and challenges. Gut. 2012:147-158

[31] Arribas JR, G.-G. J. Single (B or C), dual (BC or BD) and triple (BCD) viral hepatitis in HIV-infected patients in Madrid, Spain. AIDS. 2005:1361-1365

[32] Pineda JA, G.-G. J-G-V-M. Clinical progression of hepatitis C virus-related chronic liver disease in human immunodeficiency virus-infected patients undergoing highly active antiretroviral therapy. Hepatology. 2007;**46**:622-630

[33] Barreiro P, R.-N. S.-N.-C. Influence of liver fibrosis stage on plasma levels of antiretroviral drugs in HIV-infected patients with chronic hepatitis C. The Journal of Infectious Diseases. 2007;**195**:973-979

[34] Dolutegravir. 2018. Obtenido de http://www.ema.europa.eu/docs/es_ES/document_library/EPAR_-_Product_Information/human/002753/WC500160680.pdf [Último acceso: 25 December 2014]

[35] Etravirina. 2018. Obtenido de http://www.ema.europa.eu/docs/es_ES/document_library/

EPAR_-_Product_Information/human/000900/WC500034180.pdf [Último acceso: 25 December 2014]

[36] Ripivirina. 2018. Obtenido de http://www.ema.europa.eu/docs/es_ES/document_library/EPAR_-_Product_Information/human/002264/WC500118874.pdf [Último acceso: 25 December 2014]

[37] Hernández-Novoa B, M. A-E. Raltegravir pharmacokinetics in HIV/HCV-coinfected patients with advanced liver cirrosis (Child-Pugh C). The Journal of Antimicrobial Chemotherapy. 2014;**69**:471-475

[38] Boyd A, M.P. Effect of tenofovir with and without interferon on hepatitis D virus replication in HIV-hepatitis B virus-hepatitis D virus-infected patients. AIDS Research and Human Retroviruses. 2013:1535-1540

[39] Gotz HM, V. D. A cluster of acute hepatitis C virus infection among men who have sex with men—Results from contact tracing and public health implications. AIDS. 2005:969-974

[40] Rauch A, R M. Unsafe sex and increased incidence of hepatitis C virus infection among HIVinfected men who have sex with men: The Swiss HIV Cohort Study. Clinical Infectious Diseases. 2005:395-402

[41] Yeung LTF, K. S. Mother-to-infant transmission of hepatitis C virus. Hepatology. 2001;**34**:223-229

[42] Salmon-Ceron D, L C. Mortality 2000 Study Group. Liver disease as a major cause of death among HIV infected patients: Role of hepatitis C and B viruses and alcohol. Journal of Hepatology. 2005;799-805

[43] Bonacini M, L.S. Survival in patients with HIV infection and viral hepatitis B or C: A cohort study. AIDS. 2004;**18**:2039-2045

[44] Graham CS, B. L. Influence of human immunodeficiency virus infection on the course of hepatitis C virus infection: A meta-analysis. Clinical Infectious Diseases. 2001:562 569

[45] Rockstroh JK, M. A. Influence of hepatitis C virus infection on HIV-1 disease progression and response to highly active antiretroviral therapy. The Journal of Infectious Diseases. 2005:992-1002

[46] Weis N, L B. Impact of HCV coinfection on response to HAART and outcome in HIVinfected individuals: A nationwide cohort study. Clinical Infectious Diseases. 2006:1481-1487

[47] Bataller R, N. K. Genetic polymorphisms and the progression of liver fibrosis: A critical appraisal. Hepatology. 2003:493-503

[48] Treatment Action Group TAG. Guía sobre la hepatitis C para personas con VOH: análisis, coinfección, tratamiento y apoyo. Nueva York: Treatment Action Group TAG; 2009

[49] Welch K, M. A. Improving screening and vaccination for hepatitis B in patients coinfected with HIV and hepatitis C. The American Journal of Gastroenterology. 2002;**97**:2928-2929

[50] Rey D, K V. Increasing the number of hepatitis B vaccine injections augments anti-HBs response rate in HIV-infected patients: Effects of HIV-1 viral load. Vaccine. 2000:1161-1165

[51] Verma S, W. C. Do type and duration of antiretroviral therapy attenuate liver fibrosis in HIV-hepatitis C virus coinfected patients? Clinical Infectious Diseases. 2006;**42**:262-270

[52] Qurishi N, K C. Effect of antiretroviral therapy on liver-related mortality in patients with HIV and hepatitis C virus coinfection. Lancet. 2003:1708-1713

[53] Macías J, M J-C-G-S. Antiretroviral therapy based on protease inhibitors as a protective factor against liver fibrosis progression in patients with chronic hepatitis C. Antiviral Therapy. 2006:839-846

[54] Berenguer J, B.J. Association between exposure to nevirapine and reduced liver fibrosis progression in patients with HIV and hepatitis C virus coinfection. Clinical Infectious Diseases. 2008;**46**:137-143

[55] Sulkowski M, P S. P05411 study investigators Boceprevir versus placebo with pegylated interferon alfa-2b and ribavirin for treatment of hepatitis C virus genotype 1 in patients with HIV: A randomised, double-blind, controlled phase 2 trial. The Lancet Infectious Diseases. 2013:597-605

[56] Sulkowski MS, S. K. Combination therapy with telaprevir for chronic hepatitis C virus genotype 1 infection in patients with HIV: A randomized trial. Annals of Internal Medicine. 2013:159-186

[57] Lawitz E, M A-T. Sofosbuvir for previously untreated chronic hepatitis C infection. The New England Journal of Medicine. 2013;**368**(20):1878-1887

[58] Jensen DM, O J. Safety and Efficacy of Sofosbuvir-Containing Regimens for Hepatitis C: Real-World Experience in a Diverse, Longitudinal Observational Cohort Program and Abstracts of the 65th Annual Meeting of the American Association for the Study of Liver Diseases. Boston. 2014

[59] Dieterich D, R J. Simeprevir (TMC435) with pegylated interferon/ribavirin in patients coinfected with HCV genotype 1 and HIV-1: A phase 3 study. Clinical Infectious Diseases. 2014:1579-1587

[60] Jacobson IM, D G. Simeprevir with pegylated interferon alfa 2a plus ribavirin in treatment-naive patients with chronic hepatitis C virus genotype 1 infection (QUEST-1): A phase 3, randomised, double-blind, placebo-controlled trial. Lancet. 2014. 60494-3

[61] Manns M, M. P. Simeprevir with pegylated interferon alfa 2a or 2b plus ribavirin in treatment-naive patients with chronic hepatitis C virus genotype 1 infection (QUEST-2): A randomised, double-blind, placebo-controlled phase 3 trial. Lancet. 2014;**384**(9941):414-426

[62] Dieterich DB. Evaluation of sofosbuvir and simeprevir-based regimens in the TRIO network: Academic and community treatment of a realworld, heterogeneous population. In: Program and Abstracts of the 65th Annual Meeting of the American Association for the Study of Liver Diseases. 2014

[63] Forns X, L E. Simeprevir with peginterferon and ribavirin leads to high rates of SVR in patients with HCV genotype 1 who relapsed after previous therapy: A phase 3 trial. Gastroenterology. 2014:1669-1679

[64] Reddy KR, Z. S. Simeprevir versus telaprevir with peginterferon and ribavirin in previous null or partial responders with chronic hepatitis C virus genotype 1 infection (ATTAIN): A randomised, double blind, non-inferiority phase 3 trial. The Lancet. 2015:27-35

[65] Torriani FJ, R.-T. M.-G. Peginterferon Alfa-2a plus ribavirin for chronic hepatitis C virus infection in HIV-infected patients. The New England Journal of Medicine. 2004:438-450

[66] Laguno M, C. C. Randomized trial comparing pegylated interferon alpha-2b versus pegylated interferon alpha-2a, both plus ribavirin, to treat chronic hepatitis C in human immunodeficiency virus patients. Hepatology. 2009:22-31

[67] Van den Eynde E, C. M. Response-guided therapy for chronic hepatitis C virus infection in patients coinfected with HIV: A pilot trial. Clinical Infectious Diseases. 2009:1152-1159

[68] Rivero-Juarez A, L L-C. A 24-week treatment strategy with pegylated interferon/ribavirin in HIV/hepatitis C virus genotype 3-coinfected patients who achieved a rapid virologic response results in a high sustained virologic response rate. Clinical Infectious Diseases. 2014:130-133

[69] Zeuzem S, D. G. Sofosbuvir and ribavirin in HCV genotypes 2 and 3. The New England Journal of Medicine. 2014;**370**(21):1993-2001

[70] Sulkowski M, G D-T. Daclatasvir plus sofosbuvir for previously treated or untreated chronic HCV infection. The New England Journal of Medicine. 2014;**370**:211-212

[71] Nelson DR, C. J. All oral combination treatment with Daclatasvir (DCV) and Sofosbuvir (SOF) in patients infected with HCV genotype (GT) 3: ALLY-3 b phase 3 study. In: 65th American Association Study of Liver Diseases Annual Meeting; Boston. 2014

[72] Ruane PJ, A. D. Sofosbuvir plus ribavirin in the treatment of chronic HCV genotype 4 infection in patients of Egyptian ancestry. In: 64th Annual Meeting of the American Association for the Study of Liver Diseases. Washington. 2013

[73] Molina JM, O. C. All-oral therapy with sofosbuvir plus ribavirin for the treatment of HCV genotype 1, 2, 3 and 4 infection in patients coinfected with HIV (PHOTON-2). In: 20th International AIDS Conference, Melbourne. 2014

[74] Victrelis®. 2018. Obtenido de http://www.ema.europa.eu/docs/es_ES/document_library/EPAR__Product_Information/human/002332/WC500109786.pdf

[75] Incivo®. 2018. Available from: http://www.ema.europa.eu/docs/es_ES/document_library/EPAR__Product_Information/human/002313/WC500115529.pdf

[76] Olysio®. 2018. Obtenido de: http://ec.europa.eu/health/documents/community-register/2014/20140514128513/anx_128513_es.pdf

[77] Ouwerkerk-Mahadevan S, S V. The pharmacokinetic interactions of HCV protease inhibitor TMC435 with antiretroviral agents in healthy volunteers. In: 50th Infectious Diseases Society of America Annual Meeting; San Diego, CA. 2012

[78] Sovaldi®. 2018. Obtenido de https://www.ema.europa.eu/documents/product-information/sovaldi-epar-product-information_es.pdf

[79] Van Heeswijk RPG, B. M. Review of drug interactions with telaprevir and antiretrovirals. Antiviral Therapy. 2013;**18**:553-560

[80] Daklinza®. 2018. Available from: https://www.ema.europa.eu/documents/product-information/daklinza-epar-product-information_es.pdf

[81] Eley T, Y X. Daclatasvir: Overview of drug-drug interactions with antiretroviral agents and other common concomitant drugs. In: HIV-DART 2014, Florida. 2014. pp. 9-12

Chapter 4

Hepatitis B and C Viruses

Isaac Thom Shawa

Abstract

Hepatitis B and C viruses (HBV/HCV) are among the leading causes of liver disease. HBV is a partially double-stranded circular DNA virus whose genome is approximately 3200 bases with four overlapping open reading frames (ORFs) and belongs to *Hepadnaviridae* family. HBV prevalence varies worldwide, with high rates reported in low-income countries. Approximately 90% of HBV infections are acute, 10% progress to chronic infection among adult patients. Although HBV can be prevented by immunisation, there is no licenced HCV vaccine. HCV is a positive-sense single-stranded RNA (+ssRNA) virus belonging to Flaviviridae family. The HCV global epidemiology varies, with high prevalence rates reported in low-income countries. Approximately 80% of acutely HCV-infected individuals develop chronic hepatitis disease, while 20% resolve spontaneously. Both HBV and HCV infections can result in both acute and chronic hepatitis, ranging in severity from asymptomatic to a life-threatening disease. The HBV and HCV are transmitted through contact with contaminated blood or its products. As compared with mono-infection, HBV/HCV co-infection has higher risk of liver damage. Thus, individuals who have active HBV and HCV infections are likely to be HCV-dominant with a high HCV viral load and low or undetectable HBV DNA levels.

Keywords: viral hepatitis, hepatitis B virus, hepatitis C virus, epidemiology, pathogenesis, natural history, diagnosis, genotype, treatment, natural history

1. Hepatitis B virus

Hepatitis B virus (HBV) belongs to *Orthohepadnavirus* genus a member of the *Hepadnaviridae* family which includes other identified but less popular viruses such as *Pekin duck*, *woodchuck*, *Woolly monkey hepatitis B*, and *ground squirrel viruses*. There are some viral similarities in structure, size, nature, genetic replication, and ability to cause infection among these viruses, but HBV remains a major cause of chronic liver disease [1].

1.1 Properties

1.1.1 Structure

The HBV is a partially double stranded enveloped deoxyribonucleic acid (DNA) virus with an icosahedral symmetry that can be seen in three different forms and sizes [2]. The predominant form is a small, spherical particle (22 nm diameter), the other form has a diameter of 42 nm. Generally, the HBV virion is spherical, with a diameter of about 40–48 nm, and a length of about 3.2 kb [3]. Approximately 10^{14} HBV particles per millilitre can be present in the blood of an infected individual [4].

IntechOpen

1.1.2 HBV genome organisation

The HBV genome is made up of a circular DNA which is partly single stranded and partly double stranded. The DNA is not fully double stranded; one strand is incomplete (short strand) whereas the other forms a full length strand (complete long strand). There are small molecules that are covalently linked to the 5′ end of each HBV DNA strand. The short strand is capped with a ribonucleic acid (RNA), whereas the complete long strand is linked to a viral DNA polymerase [5]. The HBV DNA forms a circular conformation, and the full length strand together with the double stands form a short sequence of triple-stranded at the 5′ ends. The HBV envelope comprises three proteins namely; small (S), medium (M), and large (L) that are expressed on the surface of the viral particle. The S protein is the most abundant of the three. The gene S encodes for the HBV surface antigen (HBsAg) [6].

1.1.3 Genetic variation

The HBV unique life cycle requires an error-prone reverse transcriptase for replication which results in genetic variation in the form of genotypes, sub-genotypes, and mutations. The relationship between HBV genetic variation and HBV-related pathogenesis has been described which determines the outcome of HBV exposure. The HBV genome has approximately 3200 bases with four overlapping open reading frames (ORFs) namely: pre-S/S (surface proteins), pre-C/C (pre-core/core), X (transcriptional co-activator) and P (DNA polymerase) [6, 7]. The pre-S/S ORF which encodes different structural envelope proteins (large, medium and small) is contained within the P ORF, the C ORF overlaps the P ORF by a quarter of its sequence length; whereas the X ORF overlap the P ORF by a third of its sequence length. From the above mentioned four ORFs, seven different proteins are translated [6].

1.1.4 Replication cycle

The HBV replication is initiated by the attachment of the viral particles to the target cells, in this instance, hepatocytes. A number of cellular receptors such as heparin sulfate proteoglycan (HSPG), and sodium taurocholate co-transporting polypeptide (NTCP) have been reported [8]. Following attachment to the hepatocytes, the viral particles fuse with the host cell's membrane and enter the cell through endocytosis. Following penetration into the cell, the virus uncoats releasing the genetic material (HBV DNA) into the cytoplasm, which is transferred into the nucleus through nuclear pores. In the nucleus, the genetic material is converted to a complete circular double stranded DNA (dsDNA) by the action of the host DNA polymerase. The dsDNA is then transformed into a covalently closed circular DNA (cccDNA) ring (an episomal viral genome) that serves as a template for transcription of five viral RNAs [6, 9, 10]. The dsDNA is very stable and can survive in the host nucleus for a long time. The cellular RNA polymerase transcribes the negative sense single stranded DNA (−ssDNA) to form a positive sense single stranded RNA (+ssRNA). The newly transcribed positive RNA strand leaves the nucleus and migrates to the cytoplasm for protein synthesis (translation). The reverse transcriptase enzyme converts the +ssRNA to form a −ssDNA (reverse transcription). The +ssRNA is flanked by a small fragment of DNA polymerase at the 5′ end which primes the reverse transcription of ¾ of the +ssRNA but unable to complete the transcription of the remaining third. This results in the formation of dsDNA viral particles containing one partially complete strand. The mature viral particles exit the cell through budding and invade other hepatocytes and repeat the replication cycle [11–13].

1.2 Epidemiology

The HBV prevalence varies worldwide, with high rates reported in low income countries. The World Health Organisation (WHO) estimates that 6.1% of the African population, and 6.2% of the Western Pacific region are infected with HBV [1]. The HBV endemicity is heterogeneous due to variable multiple factors such as child vaccination, injection drug use, poor sensitisation campaigns among others [14].

Approximately over 250 million people are infected with HBV globally [15]. The risks of infection vary widely due to different behaviours that determine the rate of exposure. Uninfected laboratory personnel and other health-care workers are at risk of HBV exposure from infected patients, but the degree of risk depends on several factors such as the strength of their immunity, and nature of work performed [16]. Likewise, patients are also at risk from hospital staff when there are conducting their duties such as surgery, haemodialysis, and dentistry procedures.

1.3 HBV genotypes and their geographical distribution

HBV genotype plays a significant role in the clinical outcome following viral-host interaction. There are 10 different genotypes of HBV (from A to J), that determine the liver disease clinical progression, prognosis, and the response to antiviral therapy. Genotypes A, B, C, D, and F are associated with rapid progression to cirrhosis and hepatocellular carcinoma. The HBV genotypes A and B are commonly isolated in acute HBV infected individuals [17].

The HBV genotypes geographical distribution varies from one genotype and subtype to the other. The variations in the HBV genotype distributions are related to mode and route of transmission, where vertical transmissions are associated with genotypes B and C [17]. The HBV genotype A is prevalent in Africa, and North Europe; genotypes B and C are widespread in Asia; genotype D is also common in Africa, some parts of Europe, and Asia; genotype E is predominantly in West and Central Africa; genotype F is common in America; genotype G is common in Western countries; genotype H is found in Central and South America; genotype I was reported in Vietnam and Laos; while genotype J was reported in Japan [7, 18].

1.4 Transmission

The HBV cases usually occur in parenteral drug injection use through sharing of infected needles and other paraphernalia. Other risk factors include: sexual contact, transfusion of blood and/or its products, occupational exposure (e.g. laboratory, and other health-care workers, surgery, dental surgery, obstetrics and gynaecology procedures), and use of unsterile procedure when in contact with blood or body fluids. The HBV transmission routes are similar to most blood-borne viruses such as *Human immunodeficiency virus* (HIV) [7]. Transmission from mother-to-child is possible; therefore, early intervention at birth is important to protect the HBV infection. Efforts are on-going to achieve a 90% reduction in new chronic HBV infections [19].

1.5 Natural history

The natural history of chronic HBV infection (CHBV) varies and is dependent of the viral virulence factors and the host's immune response. Following exposure to HBV, some individuals (0.5–1% per year) clear the HBsAg spontaneously but remain anti-HBV positive, with undetectable HBV DNA in serum, whereas the majority progress to CHBV infection. The development of CHBV infection is determined by a complex set of interactions between the host (e.g. age, sex, immune status, and other underlying infections) and the virus (e.g. infective dose, co-infection with other viruses, and viral genotype) [20].

The CHBV infection is characterised by elevated serum alanine aminotransferase (ALT), serum HBV DNA, and/or hepatitis B e antigen (HBeAg), HBsAg which determines the phase of infection and predicts the risk of disease progression to hepatocellular carcinoma (HCC) [21]. Five CHBV phases (1, 2, 3, 4 and 5) have been described based on HBeAg, ALT, and HBV viral load [22]. Phases 1 and 2 would be HBeAg-positive, whereas phases 3 and 4 would be considered to be HBeAg-negative. The chronic HBV phase 1 is also known as immune tolerance phase (HBeAg-positive chronic HBV infection), phase 2 (immune clearance phase or HBeAg-positive chronic hepatitis B), phase 3 (inactive carrier phase or HBeAg-negative chronic HBV infection), phase 4 (reactivation phase or HBeAg-negative chronic hepatitis B), and phase 5 (occult HBV infection or HBsAg-negative phase). During the early stages of CHBV infection, the serum ALT levels are normal or slightly elevated whereas the HBV DNA, and hepatitis B e antigen (HBeAg) levels are elevated in serum. This first stage is followed by a second phase where the HBeAg, HBsAg, and ALTs are elevated. After varying intervals, the ALT levels return to normal, and the HBV DNA reach undetectable levels or suppressed to low levels, resulting in an inactive HBV carrier state. The fourth phase is characterised by fluctuation of HBV diagnostic markers that include HBV DNA, ALTs and HBV antibody concentrations [21, 22]. The fifth phase is characterised by the presence of anti-HBc antibodies, absence of HBsAg, detectable or undetectable anti-HBs antibodies. Of note, not all HBV patients fit into these phases of disease progression. Chronic HBV infection does not always represent development of chronic hepatitis B disease. Thus, not all patients with HBV infection have hepatitis disease [22].

1.6 Clinical features

The possible outcome following HBV exposure depend on series of complex mechanisms that could lead to spontaneous clearance with detectable HBV antibodies, or establishment of chronic HBV infection (described in four phases). The HBV incubation period varies greatly often about 2–6 months, but shorter incubation periods have been observed related to high infective doses. Symptoms of HBV infection may include fever, nausea, vomiting, abdominal pain, dark urine, anorexia, myalgia, and jaundice (is the hallmark of severe liver disease). In some cases, arthralgia may occur, hepatocellular damage may be detected [7, 21].

1.7 Pathogenesis

1.7.1 Acute infection

It is estimated that approximately 90% of HBV infections are acute, where about 10% progress to chronic HBV infection among adult patients, whereas 30–50% for infection among under-5 children. The HBV replicates in hepatocytes following successful entry into the cell by binding the host cellular receptors. In acute infection before seroconversion, the HBV viral load is high before the host immune response kicks in. The viral markers such HBeAg, and HBeAg are expressed on the host cellular cytoplasmic membrane that trigger an adaptive immune response (both B and T cells) [6, 23].

Within hours following HBV exposure, the host innate immune response by releasing the interferon-α which modulate the immune system, and has a direct antiviral effect [24]. This is followed by a transient release of interleukin (IL)-6 to control the viral spread and virus-induced cellular apoptosis. The production of interferons and other cytokines enhances the expression of major histocompatibility complex class I (MHC-I) that recognises the viral antigens which leads to lysis of infected hepatocytes. The subsequent activation of natural killer (NK) and cytotoxic killer cells may reduce the HBV viral load through secretion of different cytokines, which may lead to hepatocellular damage. An anti-inflammatory cytokine IL-10 suppresses the activation of NK T cells. The liver damage is less severe in the HBV acute infection [25–27].

1.7.2 Chronic infection

HBV persistence and development of chronic HBV infection is a result of neonatal tolerance to HBV if acquired vertically. The HBV precore antigen, HBeAg which crosses the placenta is able to induce neonatal tolerance to HBV ex vivo. The HBV adult infections have a low rate (<5%) of developing chronic HBV infection as compared to neonates. However, the mechanism that contributes to inadequate immune response a key feature of onset of chronic HBV in adults is unclear.

Of note, nearly 15–40% of HBV infected individuals are at risk of developing cirrhosis during their life time, and nearly 5% risk of HCC with cirrhosis. During the immune clearance phase (phase 2), the viral load is reduced due to the action of the cytotoxic T cells that destroy the infected hepatocytes. Since the action of NK and cytotoxic T cells in chronic HBV infection is inefficient, the destruction of hepatocytes happens for years which increases the possibility of reinfection [11, 15, 25, 26, 28].

The production of different HBV specific antibodies such as those against HBeAg, HBcAg, and HBsAg prevent the spreading of viral particles between hepatocytes. Ineffective viral suppression could lead to cirrhosis which is a prime factor for carcinogenesis. The integration of viral and host genome, and the formation of cccDNA during viral replication are essential steps towards development of hepatic carcinogenesis. Both B and T cell responses to HBcAg could be suppressed by secretion of some HBV antigens such as HBeAg, which results in inhibition of HBcAg-specific T cells to eliminate HBV infected hepatocytes. Likewise, increased levels of HBsAg also suppress the immune elimination of infected cells [9–11].

Increased risks of cirrhosis and HCC are associated with male gender, race, HIV, hepatitis C virus (HCV) co-infection, persistence of increased HBV viral load (high HBV DNA levels), HBeAg negative status, elevated ALTs, and the general impairment of host immune responses.

The HBV clinical outcomes are classified into: immune-tolerant, immune clearance, inactive and recovery phase. Occult HBV infection is a phenomenon that occurs in patients who receive HBV vaccine and/or hepatitis B immunoglobulin injection who may develop chronic HBV infection with PreS and/or S gene mutations. In these four clinical stages of HBV infection, the HBV DNA levels are high in immune tolerance and immune clearance stages, and become undetectable in inactive phase. HBV isolated from chemotherapy of immunocompromised patients show mutations in the PreS, S, basal core promoter (BCP) or Pre-C regions (**Figure 1**) (Adapted from [6]).

1.8 Laboratory diagnosis

1.8.1 Acute HBV infection

Nearly 90% of acute HBV infections in adults are self-limiting, with only a small proportion (<1%) progress to severe acute infection. Acute HBV infection presents with non-specific signs and symptoms. The HBV incubation period may be 6 weeks or more following exposure. Some of the signs and symptoms of acute HBV infection may include: malaise, fever, nausea, dark urine and anorexia. The majority of acute HBV infected individual are usually asymptomatic with elevated levels

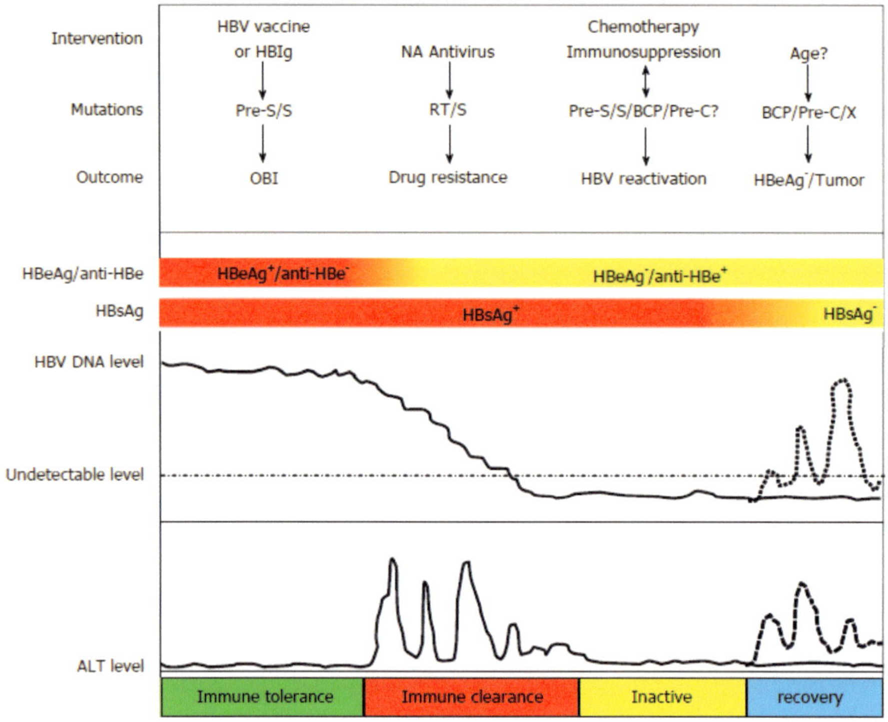

Figure 1.
HBV pathogenesis and clinical outcomes.

of ALT, total bilirubin, and total protein. The HBsAg positive test suggest an HBV infection, however it is advisable to repeat the test after 6 months to determine HBV spontaneous resolution or establishment of chronic infection [29].

1.8.2 Chronic HBV infection

The majority of acute HBV infected individuals clear the infection spontaneously, whereas 5–10% progress to develop chronic HBV infection. The majority of chronic HBV infected individuals are at risk of developing chronic active disease (HBV hepatitis) which may progress to cirrhosis and hepatocellular carcinoma. The development of chronic HBV infection does not follow clinical phases (1–5) in sequential order as described above. The HBV diagnostic markers vary from one clinical phase to another.

1.8.2.1 Immune-tolerance phase

During the immune-tolerance phase of chronic HBV infection, the virus is actively replicating, but there is a reduced inflammation response. The individuals who get HBV infection at birth stay in this phase for decades before progressing to the next phases of liver disease. The laboratory diagnosis markers that characterise the immune-tolerance phase include: increased HBV viral load (>million copies IU/ml), normal ALT, HBsAg positive test [22, 30].

1.8.2.2 Immune clearance phase

During the immune-active phase, the virus continues to replicate and cause noticeable liver damage. The host immune response activates the signalling cascade that leads to inflammatory response, leading to liver fibrosis. The individuals who were HBV susceptible during childhood stay in this phase for decades but clinical feature manifest in mid-thirties. During this stage, the laboratory diagnostic features fluctuate from HBeAg positive to negative, with detectable anti-HBe antibodies. Classic HBV immune-active phase is characterised by the HBeAg seroconversion and detection of different anti- HBV immunoglobulins. The HBeAg seroconversion is associated with reduced disease progression rate to development of cirrhosis and end stage liver disease. The laboratory detection markers include: increased ALT levels, four-fold increase in HBV viral load, positive HBeAg, and liver fibrosis [22].

1.8.2.3 Inactive carrier phase

In this phase, the anti-HBe antibodies are detectable, whereas the ALT levels return to normal, and HBV viral load is suppressed and may be undetectable. The extent of liver damage depends on an inflammatory immune response, but liver fibrosis is noticeable if it was observed in the previous stage of liver disease. The majority (nearly 80%) of chronic HBV infected patients remain in this stage whereas nearly 20% may revert to the immune-tolerance phase. Some of the laboratory diagnostic markers of this stage include: Normal ALT, negative HBeAg, reduced or undetectable HBV viral load (<2000 copies IU/ml), and variable liver fibrosis [22].

1.8.2.4 Reactivation phase

This phase is also known as the immune reactivation phase where the chronic HBV is very active with detectable anti-HBe antibodies. Some of the diagnostic markers include: increased HBV viral load, elevated ALT, negative HBeAg, moderate-to-severe liver fibrosis, sometimes cirrhosis, and hepatocellular carcinoma. In this phase, people have seroconverted to anti-HBe positive, but their chronic HBV is very active. The ALT levels and HBV viral load are elevated. The liver inflammation and fibrosis levels are moderate to severe [22].

1.8.2.5 Occult HBV infection

This phase is also known as HBsAg-negative phase. During this phase the viral detection markers such as HBsAg, anti-HBs, and HBV DNA are usually negative. The anti-HBc antibodies are positive, and in rare cases, the anti-HBs could be positive. The serum ALT levels are usually normal, with detectable cccDNA copies [22].

1.9 Treatment, prevention, and control

The treatment and management efforts of HBV infection are aimed at reducing the incidence rates, prevent development of chronic HBV disease, progression to HCC, and obviously death from HBV-related liver disease. The decision to treat is based on clinical assessment of phases of HBV infection based primarily on the biochemical, virological, serological investigations, and the stage of liver disease [22].

Historically, the interferon-based therapy has been the principal treatment option for HBV infection. The current HBV treatment guidelines recommend treating patients with increased viral load, decompensated liver cirrhosis, and HCC. Treatment is less favourable in HBV infected individuals classified as belonging to first phase chronic HBV infection. The recommended standard treatment for HBV infection is the nucleoside analogues (NAs) and/or IFN-based therapy. The response to IFN-based therapy is robust which results in loss of HBeAg and HBsAg as opposed to NA monotherapy. However, IFN is less efficient at suppressing viral replication and is reported to be associated with adverse effects compared to the NAs. The IFN-α has a direct antiviral effect through inhibition of viral assembly [8, 31].

The pegylated IFN-α administered parenterally, and the NAs (Entecavir and Tenofovir) are the first line antiviral drugs recommended for chronic HBV treatment. These drugs are hardly available in low income countries due to high costs. The most widely antiviral drug for HBV treatment is lamivudine which is a nucleoside analogue that inhibits the synthesis of HBV DNA ex vivo. The lamivudine course has resulted in a marked reduction in viral DNA, normal ALT levels, HBeAg-positive cases seroconverting to become anti-HBe positive. Other antiviral drugs that have been used to treat HBV infection include adefovir, emtricitabine, telbivudine, and clevudine. For end stage liver disease such as HCC, liver transplantation is recommended. There is an urgent need to develop alternative HBV therapeutic agents that can successfully suppress HBV replication and decrease the risk of disease progression to fibrosis and HCC [8, 31].

Several approaches can be employed for the prevention and control of HCV infection. Screening of blood donations has significantly reduced the risks of HBV transmission through transfusion of blood and/or its products [32]. Modification of risk behaviours proves to be an effective measure to prevent HBV transmission. Some essential approaches include voiding contact with blood and body fluids, practicing safe sexual contact, avoiding drug use (either injecting or snorting), and use of sterile needles when body piercing and acupunctures. The implementation of health and safety policies that include wearing personal protective equipment when performing risky procedures in the hospital or during accidents and emergencies [22].

Herd immunity can be provided through incorporation of HBV vaccine in the child immunisation schedule. Other important approaches to prevent HBV infection include: antenatal screening for identification of carrier mothers, and universal infant and adolescent vaccination. If universal vaccination is not implemented yet, HBV vaccine should be given to other groups at special risk of HBV exposure.

1.10 Vaccination

Hepatitis B is a vaccine preventable disease. In 1965, Dr. Baruch Blumberg and his team discovered the HBV vaccine which prevents the establishment of HBV infection and liver cancer [33].

1.10.1 Active immunisation

The current HBV vaccine is given in three doses as follows: first dose given within 24 hours, second dose given 1 month later, and a third booster dose given at 6 months of age. The HBV vaccine elicits humoral immune response that is mediated by secreted anti-HBs antibodies. Such an antibody-mediated response is influenced by several factors including age, sex, immune status, and underlined pathological conditions. High seroconversion rates of >90% are seen in young female adults as opposed to their male counterparts or older men, whereas lower rates are observed in immunosuppressed individuals [34].

The HBV vaccine was made available since 1982. In 1991, the WHO recommended that each country adopt and implement universal HBV vaccination programme. HBV vaccine is included in the new-born immunisation schedule where first dose is given shortly after birth, second dose at 1–2 months of age, and third dose at 6–18 months of age. A child born to a HBV-positive mother should receive the HBV vaccine and HBIG combination as early as within 12 hours after birth to protect baby from HBV infection. The vaccine may cause swelling, soreness and redness on the site of injection, and a mild fever [35, 36].

1.10.2 Passive immunisation

The plasma-derived hepatitis B vaccine was licenced for human use in 1981. Hepatitis B immunoglobulin (HBIG) is an anti-HBs prepared from plasma of donors with high titres of antibodies of the HBsAg. The administration of anti-HBV immunoglobulins induces an adaptive immune response. Since the HBIG contains anti-HBV immunoglobulins, it offers an immediate short-term protection in risk population who have not yet received HBV vaccine. The HBIG half-life is estimated at 3 weeks, but long-term protection can be achieved by a combination of HBIG and HBV vaccine at the time of HBIG initial administration. Therefore, an HBIG booster dose is not necessary when a HBV vaccine is administered concurrently with HBIG [37, 38]. The HBIG dose of 300–500 IU in 3 ml is administered either intramuscularly (IM) or intravenously as a post-exposure prophylaxis, given to babies born to infected mothers, or prevention of the establishment of chronic HBV infection in liver transplants. HBIG should be administered 24–48 hours after a potential exposure to HBV, and a second dose 4 weeks later. An absolute protection against HBV is unlikely to be achieved but a vaccine efficacy of 76% has been reported, and the protection could last for at least 22 years [38]. In babies, a 6 month course of HBIG is initiated that offers nearly 70% efficacy. High rates (nearly 90%) are achieved when combining HBIG and HBV vaccine.

The HBIG side effects include allergic reactions, back pain, muscle pain, nausea, and general body pain.

1.10.3 Who should get vaccinated?

HBV vaccination is aimed at preventing HBV transmission to uninfected individuals, and ultimately eradicating the virus from the population. A small subset of HBV exposed individuals exist who have persistent HBV infection, could have undetectable or carry low levels of the HBV DNA; and are termed 'inactive HBV carriers.' The HBV carrier state is a potential reservoir for HBV transmission through contact with the infected body fluids.

The HBV vaccination is recommended in the following [16]:

- Newly born babies who could become long-term HBV carriers if not protected immediately after birth
- Commercial sex workers
- Intravenous drug users
- Occupational exposures (health care workers, laboratory personnel, Medical personnel, dental therapists, first aid providers)
- Anyone who comes in contact with infected blood
- Victims of sexual assault

The passive and active HBV immunisation is 95% effective in preventing establishment of chronic infection, but HBV reinfection is possible following continuous exposure to the virus.

2. Hepatitis C virus

Hepatitis C virus (HCV) belongs to the Flaviviridae family and the genus *Hepacivirus* [39]; and has evolved over hundreds and thousands of years with human as the only host. When HCV was first identified in 1989 [40] as the aetiological agent of non-A/non-B hepatitis the extent of the global health problem from HCV related cirrhosis and hepatocellular carcinoma was underestimated. Today HCV remains a global public health problem with a prevalence at 2.8%, with relatively low prevalence in Europe (0.6–5.6%), with pockets of high prevalence in Africa (Egypt has the highest prevalence rate estimated at 14% based on anti-HCV antibody testing) [41].

2.1 Discovery

HCV was discovered in 1989 [40]. It was thought to be the primary cause of transfusion-associated non-A/non-B hepatitis (NANBH). Following intensive search through development of different immunological and serological assays, an experimental chimpanzee model was utilised to identify the presence of an NANBH transmissible agent. Immunoscreening of bacterial complementary deoxyribonucleic acid (cDNA) obtained from chimpanzee blood samples that were infected with NANBH enabled the isolation of a single cDNA clone, and the translation of viral proteins was possible. On 21st April 1989, Michael Houghton and his colleagues in collaboration with Daniel Bradley announced the discovery of NANBH aetiological agent and named it '*Hepatitis C virus*' [40].

2.2 Properties

2.2.1 Structure

HCV is a small, enveloped virus that contains two viral glycoproteins expressed on the surface of the virus particle namely, E1 and E2 [42, 43]. The HCV is a positive-sense single-stranded RNA (+ssRNA) virus that has approximately 10,000 bases in length. Visualised viral particles are estimated to be between 40 and 60 nm [44]. The HCV gene sequence contains a single long open reading frame (ORF) that produces large polyprotein precursor of more than 3000 amino acids. The HCV ORF is flanked by 5′ and 3′ non-translated regions (NTRs). During and after translation, the polyprotein precursor is cleaved by the proteases for synthesis of mature structural and non-structural (NS) proteins [45].

2.2.2 Lipoviral particle

The hepatic portal vein and hepatic arteries circulate blood through the liver. The HCV particles circulating in the blood stream are reported to bind directly to low density lipoprotein (LDL), very low density lipoprotein (VLDL), chylomicrons, different types of apolipoproteins (apo) [46, 47]. The lipoviral particles (LVPs) are highly infectious viral particles that form a complex with VLDL composed of triglyceride-rich, and cholesterol-rich lipoproteins that are believed to contain apoA1, apoB, apoC1, and apoE [48, 49]. During the LVPs formation they also form a complex with viral envelope glycoproteins E1 and E2; and nucleocapsids [50–52]. It is believed that the LVPs facilitate the viral attachment and entry into the target host cell [53].

Figure 2 shows an HCV viral particle in association with lipoproteins in a structure termed 'lipoviral particle.' The viral envelope glycoproteins E1, and E2

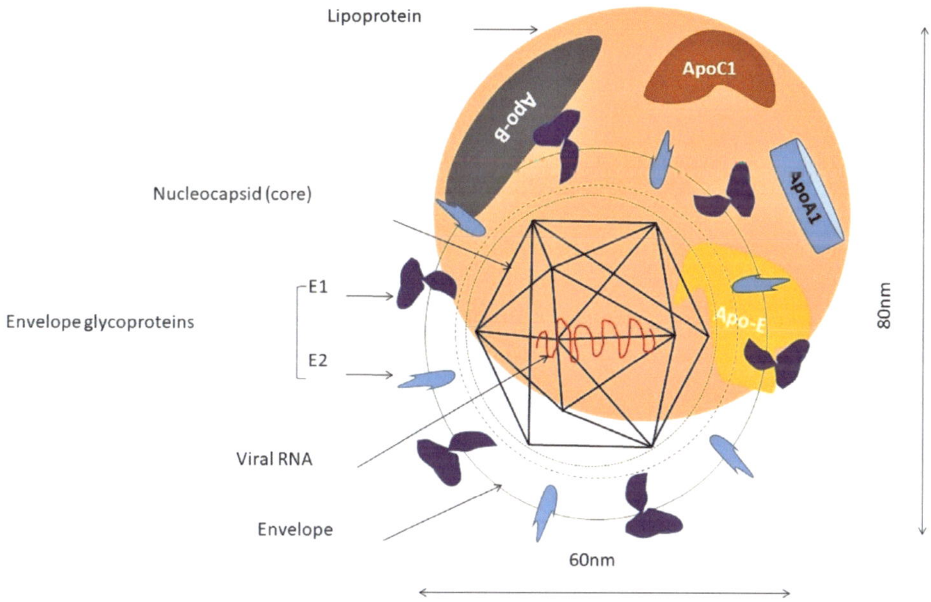

Figure 2.
Hepatitis C virus lipoviral structure.

help to attach the virus to the host cell receptors. The apolipoprotein components of the LVPs are also facilitate viral binding via cellular lipoprotein receptors. (Adapted from https://pearl.plymouth.ac.uk/handle/10026.1/10386).

2.2.3 Replication

The primary in vivo target of HCV replication are hepatocytes, however, lack of small animal model to propagate HCV hampers efforts to fully describe the HCV replication.

Following the formation of LVPs in vascular compartment, they travel to the liver for attachment to the hepatocytes utilising the viral envelope glycoproteins, and the lipoprotein plasma lipoproteins component of the LVPs. The HCV LVP levels determine viral persistence [54]. The viral particles utilise the virally encoded envelope glycoproteins E1 and E2, and different classes of apolipoproteins (apoA-1, apoB, apoC-1 and apoE) to bind to host cellular receptors, co-receptors, and entry factors to facilitate viral entry into the cell cytoplasm [53]. Some of the reported host cellular receptors and entry factors include: tetraspanin CD81, highly sulphated glycosaminoglycans (HS-GAGs) [55], low density lipoprotein receptor (LDLR), and Scavenger receptor class B type I (SR-BI) [56]. The viral entry involves clathrin-mediated endocytosis, and membrane fusion.

After entry, the viral RNA genome is translated for production of different viral proteins in endoplasmic reticulum (ER). Translation is of the polyprotein from HCV RNA is an essential first step after releasing the viral genetic material into the host cytoplasm. Since the HCV RNA is a positive-sense single strand, it directly serves as a template for translation. The 5′ NTR serves as the primary site where HCV RNA translation into polypeptides is initiated which results in expression of structural and NS viral proteins (NS1, 2, 3, 4 and 5) required for genome replication [52].

Several HCV NS proteins such as NS3/4A, NS4B, NS5A, and NS5B form part of a complex replication machinery which replicate a positive-sense RNA genome through a negative-sense RNA intermediate which takes place in lipid droplets (LDs) [57]. The HCV replication process occurs in specialised membranous web on the endoplasmic reticulum membrane. Initiation of assembly of viral proteins requires release of viral genomes from the membranous web to the cytosolic site of the ER. Therefore, progeny viral assembly initiates in the cytosol followed by maturation and release of the viral particles on the lumenal side of the ER membrane. During this process, the virions become lipidated through further interaction with the host lipid components, transported through the Golgi apparatus. After budding, the viral particles are transported to the extracellular environment through the lipid secretory channels [58].

2.3 HCV epidemiology, genotypes, and global distribution

HCV is one of the major causes of liver disease globally. Over the years HCV prevalence rates have increased to 2.8% worldwide, where an estimated 71 million people are reported to have chronic hepatitis C infection [59]. The World Health Organisation (WHO) estimates that nearly 399,000 people die annually due to HCV related liver disease. The HCV global distribution varies with high prevalence rates reported among people who inject drugs (PWIDs) [60]. Egypt has the highest burden of HCV infection due to use of non-sterile injecting needles during the mass treatment of schistosomiasis. In the 80s, the tartar emeric treatment was replaced by an oral drug, praziquantel for treatment of schistosomiasis [41].

Seven major HCV genotypes (1–7) were reported that comprise different subspecies [61]. Determination of HCV genotypes is essential and predicts the disease outcome, and treatment options. Globally, HCV genotype 1 is the most prevalence, followed by genotypes 3, 2, and 4. Genotypes 1, 2, and 3 have a worldwide distribution but predominantly highly prevalent in western countries [62, 63]. Genotype 4 is prevalent in Egypt and the middle-east, genotype 5 is prevalent in South Africa, and genotype is high in Hongkong. Genotype 6 is endemic in Southeast Asia [64, 65], whereas genotype 7 is was reported in central Africa [66].

The HCV nucleotide sequences show some genetic differences from one genotype to another. Genotypes show nearly 30% sequence diversity from each other [30, 67].

2.4 Transmission

HCV is primarily transmitted via parenteral exposure to the virus, though sometimes it can be transmitted sexually. Injection drug use (IDU) remains the highest risk factor for HCV infection in western countries. Some of the risk factors for HCV transmission include: blood transfusion before initiation of universal donor screening programme in 1991 [68], occupational exposure, tattooing, organ transplant from an infected donor, acupunctures, haemodialysis, and use of unsterilized razor blades and other paraphernalia for cultural rituals. Some studies have reported vertical transmission, as well as cell-to-cell transmission. The frequency of mother-to-child transmission is estimated at between 3 and 10% in some studies. The following factors have not been described to transmit HCV; hugging, kissing, hand shake, and/or sharing drinking bottles with an infected person [69].

2.5 HCV natural history

Exposure to HCV usually results in an asymptomatic acute HCV infection which is followed by three possible outcomes: clearance of the virus spontaneously

(15–25%), progression to chronic HCV infection (>80%), or remain uninfected without detectable HCV RNA and anti-HCV antibodies [70–72].

2.5.1 Acute HCV infection

Diagnosis of acute HCV infection is problematic because the majority of infected individuals are asymptomatic with only 20–30% go on to develop clinical signs and symptoms. An acute infection occurs during the first 6 months following exposure, and during this period few infected individuals complain of fever, fatigue, nausea, anorexia, vomiting, and sometimes mild jaundice appears [73].

The HCV incubation period ranges from 3 to 12 weeks. The development of clinical manifestations depends on multiple viral and host factors that may include: infective dose (viral load), viral genotype, route of transmission, gender, age, and host immune response among others. HCV seroconversion window period ranges between 8 and 12 weeks after viremia. Of note, acute HCV infection does not always lead to the development of chronic infection. Nearly 20% of acute HCV infected individuals resolve the infection spontaneously with detectable anti-HCV antibodies, but without HCV RNA [73].

2.5.2 Chronic HCV infection

Following the establishment of acute HCV infection, nearly 80% of infected individuals progress to develop chronic HCV infection. Persistent HCV infection is usually associated with progressive hepatitis disease, with detectable HCV RNA and anti-HCV antibodies. Despite detection of HCV markers in the blood, there is no correlation between viremia and disease severity. The majority of chronically infected individuals develop fibrosis, cirrhosis and hepatocellular carcinoma (usually after 20 or more years followed infection) if no antiviral treatment is initiated. Once cirrhosis develops, the situation is usually irreversible but further liver damage can be prevented with early diagnosis and treatment. The development of cirrhosis and HCC is accelerated by immunosuppression [74]. Chronic HCV infection causes several histological changes in the liver and classifies the disease into persistent HCV infection, and active HCV infection with or without cirrhosis.

HCV infected individuals do not realise that they are infected, until the following signs and symptoms appear: anorexia, vomiting, fever, dark urine, jaundice, weight loss, and myalgia.

2.6 Laboratory diagnosis

Since seroconversion takes 8–12 weeks after viremia, serological diagnosis of acute HCV infection is tricky. During the acute stage, molecular diagnostic methods are reliable where HCV RNA can be detected within 1–3 weeks after exposure. Anti-HCV antibodies can be detected at the onset of clinical signs and symptoms. The HCV laboratory diagnostic methods include detection of specific anti-HCV antibodies, quantification of HCV RNA, and characterisation of HCV biomarkers. Enzyme immunoassay (EIA), rapid diagnostic kits, and polymerase chain reaction (PCR) techniques are commonly used for HCV diagnosis. It is prudent that each facility should establish a testing algorithm that includes screening, supplementary, and confirmatory testing methods. Detection of HCV RNA confirms active infection, whereas detection of anti-HCV antibodies suggests clearance of HCV infection spontaneously or establishment of chronic infection. It is advisable to confirm all anti-HCV positive test results with a nucleic acid test to rule-out spontaneous viral clearance [75]. Once chronic infection has been noted, further liver damage has to be assessed by performing liver function tests, liver biopsy, or other non-invasive procedures. In chronic HCV infection, the following markers are elevated: alanine transaminase (ALT), aspartate transaminase (AST), alkaline phosphatase (ALP), total protein (TP), gamma-glutamyl transpeptidase (GGT), prothrombin time (PT), total bilirubin, and sometimes a fasting serum acid [76].

2.7 Treatment, prevention, and control

For the past few decades, the standard HCV treatment has been interferon based therapy but there were increased cases of adverse effects, and reduced sustained viral response rate (50%). It is not all HCV cases that require treatment, since some individuals are asymptomatic. When treatment is desirable, the primary goal is cure [77]. The arrival of direct acting antivirals (DAAs) since 2014 with a high rate of responses to this treatment has brought a great expectancy of the possible cure and eradication of HCV infection in the next future. The WHO recommends sofosbuvir, daclatasvir, and the sofosbuvir/ledipasvir combination that has a 95% reported cure rate. Detection of the HCV genotypes and subtypes is relevant to response to the DAAs. The DAAs disrupt viral replication which subsequent establishment of HCV infection [78]. The following classes of DAAs have been suggested: NS3/4A protease inhibitors, NS5A inhibitors, NS5B nucleoside polymerase (NS5B RNA-dependent RNA polymerase) inhibitors, and NS5B non-nucleoside polymerase inhibitors. The DAAs have reduced the treatment duration (12 weeks to achieve cure), changed the drug administration route, reduced adverse effects, improved efficacy, viral sustained response, and tolerability [30]. Access to DAAs is still limited in low income countries, but the introduction of generic versions of DAAs has reduced the production and consumption cost in low income countries. It is estimated that HCV viremic burden will decline by approximately 60% [79].

Author details

Isaac Thom Shawa
Faculty of Biomedical Science and Health Professions, University of Malawi College of Medicine, Blantyre, Malawi

*Address all correspondence to: ishawa@medcol.mw

References

[1] Chisari FV, Isogawa M, Wieland SF. Pathogenesis of Hepatitis B virus infection. Pathologie et Biologie. 2010,58.258-266. DOI. 10.1016/j.patbio.2009.11.001.Pathogenesis

[2] Gilbert RJC, Beales L, Blond D, Simon MN, Lin BY, Chisari FV, et al. Hepatitis B small surface antigen particles are octahedral. In: Proceedings of the National Academy of Sciences. 2005. DOI: 10.1073/pnas.0505062102

[3] Hu J, Liu K. Complete and incomplete hepatitis B virus particles: Formation, function, and application. Viruses. 2017. DOI: 10.3390/v9030056

[4] Shih C, Yang CC, Choijilsuren G, Chang CH, Liou AT. Hepatitis B virus. Trends in Microbiology. 2018. DOI: 10.1016/j.tim.2018.01.009

[5] Zhang ZH, Wu CC, Chen XW, Li X, Li J, Lu MJ. Genetic variation of hepatitis B virus and its significance for pathogenesis. World Journal of Gastroenterology. 2016;**22**:126-144. DOI: 10.3748/wjg.v22.i1.126

[6] Lin CL, Kao JH. Natural history of acute and chronic hepatitis B: The role of HBV genotypes and mutants. Best Practice & Research. Clinical Gastroenterology. 2017;**31**:249-255. DOI: 10.1016/j.bpg.2017.04.010

[7] Lok AS, Zoulim F, Dusheiko G, Ghany MG. Hepatitis B cure: From discovery to regulatory approval. Hepatology. 2017;**66**:1296-1313. DOI: 10.1002/hep.29323

[8] Locarnini S, Zoulim F. Molecular genetics of HBV infection. Antiviral Therapy. 2010. DOI: 10.3851/IMP1619

[9] Testoni B, Durantel D, Zoulim F. Novel targets for hepatitis B virus therapy. Liver International. 2017. DOI: 10.1111/liv.13307

[10] Seeger C, Mason WS. Molecular biology of hepatitis B virus infection. Virology. 2015. DOI: 10.1016/j.virol.2015.02.031

[11] Frentzen A, Anggakusuma GE, Hueging K, Knocke S, Ginkel C, et al. Cell entry, efficient RNA replication, and production of infectious hepatitis C virus progeny in mouse liver-derived cells. Hepatology. 2014. DOI: 10.1002/hep.26626

[12] Blondot ML, Bruss V, Kann M. Intracellular transport and egress of hepatitis B virus. Journal of Hepatology. 2016. DOI: 10.1016/j.jhep.2016.02.008

[13] World Health Organization. Hepatitis B. WHO. 2018. https://www.who.int/news-room/fact-sheets/detail/hepatitis-b [Accessed: 02 January 2019]

[14] Zampino R, Boemio A, Sagnelli C, Alessio L, Adinolfi LE, Sagnelli E, et al. Hepatitis B virus burden in developing countries. World Journal of Gastroenterology. 2015;**21**:11941-11953. DOI: 10.3748/wjg.v21.i42.11941

[15] Tsai KN, Kuo CF, Ou JHJ. Mechanisms of Hepatitis B virus persistence. Trends in Microbiology. 2018. DOI: 10.1016/j.tim.2017.07.006

[16] Nelson NP, Easterbrook PJ, McMahon BJ. Epidemiology of Hepatitis B virus infection and impact of vaccination on disease. Clinics in Liver Disease. 2016. DOI: 10.1016/j.cld.2016.06.006

[17] Sunbul M. Hepatitis B virus genotypes: Global distribution and clinical importance. World Journal of Gastroenterology. 2014. DOI: 10.3748/wjg.v20.i18.5427

[18] Ott JJ, Stevens GA, Groeger J, Wiersma ST. Global epidemiology of Hepatitis B virus infection: New

estimates of age-specific HBsAg seroprevalence and endemicity. Vaccine. 2012;**30**:2212-2219. DOI: 10.1016/j.vaccine.2011.12.116

[19] Nayagam S, Thursz M, Sicuri E, Conteh L, Wiktor S, Low-Beer D, et al. Requirements for global elimination of hepatitis B: A modelling study. The Lancet Infectious Diseases. 2016;**16**:1399-1408. DOI: 10.1016/S1473-3099(16)30204-3

[20] Chang MH. Hepatitis B virus infection. In: Suchy FJ, Sokol RJ, Balistreri WF, editors. Liver Disease in Children. 4th ed. Cambridge, England, UK: Cambridge University Press; 2014. pp. 176-294. DOI: 10.1017/CBO9781139012102.019

[21] Liaw YF. Natural history of chronic hepatitis B virus infection. In: Thomas HC, ASF L, editors. Viral Hepatitis. 4th ed. Hoboken, New Jersey, USA: Wiley; 2013. pp. 143-153. DOI: 10.1002/9781118637272.ch10

[22] Lampertico P, Agarwal K, Berg T, Buti M, Janssen HLA, Papatheodoridis G, et al. EASL 2017 Clinical Practice Guidelines on the management of hepatitis B virus infection. Journal of Hepatology. 2017. DOI: 10.1016/j.jhep.2017.03.021

[23] Bowden S. Hepatitis B virus. In: Carter IW, Schuller M, James GS, Sloots TP, Halliday CL, editors. PCR for Clinical Microbiology: An Australian and International Perspective Illustrate. Berlin, Germany: Springer Science & Business Media; 2010. DOI: 10.1007/978-90-481-9039-3_36

[24] Wang FS, Shi JJ. Immunopathogenesis of hepatitis B virus (HBV) infection. In: Kao J-H, Chen D-S, editors. Hepatitis B Virus and Liver Disease. Singapore: Springer; 2018. pp. 45-62. DOI: 10.1007/978-981-10-4843-2_3

[25] Baumert TF, Thimme R, von Weizsäcker F. Pathogenesis of hepatitis B virus infection. World Journal of Gastroenterology. 2007. DOI: 10.3748/wjg.v13.i1.82

[26] Ferrari C. HBV and the immune response. Liver International. 2015. DOI: 10.1111/liv.12749

[27] Busca A, Kumar A. Innate immune responses in hepatitis B virus (HBV) infection. Virology Journal. 2014. DOI: 10.1186/1743-422X-11-22

[28] Tawar RG, Colpitts CC, Timm J, Fehm T, Roggendorf M, Meisel H, et al. Acute hepatitis C virus infection induces anti-host cell receptor antibodies with virus-neutralizing properties. Hepatology. 2015;**62**:726-736. DOI: 10.1002/hep.27906

[29] Cornberg M, Wong VWS, Locarnini S, Brunetto M, Janssen HLA, Chan HLY. The role of quantitative hepatitis B surface antigen revisited. Journal of Hepatology. 2017. DOI: 10.1016/j.jhep.2016.08.009

[30] Razavi H, Robbins S, Zeuzem S, Negro F, Buti M, Duberg AS, et al. Hepatitis C virus prevalence and level of intervention required to achieve the WHO targets for elimination in the European Union by 2030: A modelling study. The Lancet Gastroenterology & Hepatology. 2017;**2**:325-336. DOI: 10.1016/S2468-1253(17)30045-6

[31] Kwon HK, Lok ASF. Treatment of hepatitis B. In: Thomas HC, Lok ASF, Locarnini SA, Zuckerman AJ, editors. Viral Hepatitis. 4th ed., Hoboken, New Jersey, USA: Wiley; 2013. pp. 188-202. DOI: 10.1002/9781118637272.ch14.

[32] Dwyre DM, Holland PV. Hepatitis viruses. In: Barbara JAJ, Regan FAM, Contreras M, editors. Transfusion Microbiology. Cambridge, England, UK: Cambridge University Press;

2008. pp. 9-24. DOI: 10.1017/CBO9780511545245.005

[33] Gerlich WH. Medical virology of hepatitis B: How it began and where we are now. Virology Journal. 2013;**10**:239. DOI: 10.1186/1743-422X-10-239

[34] Bonanni P, Pesavento G, Bechini A, Tiscione E, Mannelli F, Benucci C, et al. Impact of universal vaccination programmes on the epidemiology of hepatitis B: 10 years of experience in Italy. Vaccine. 2003. DOI: 10.1016/S0264-410X(02)00580-7

[35] Mangen MJJ, Stibbe H, Urbanus A, Siedenburg EC, Waldhober Q, de Wit GA, et al. Targeted outreach hepatitis B vaccination program in high-risk adults: The fundamental challenge of the last mile. Vaccine. 2017. DOI: 10.1016/j.vaccine.2017.04.068

[36] Centers for Disease Control and Prevention. Hepatitis B vaccination—United States, 1982-2002. Morbidity and Mortality Weekly Report. 2002

[37] Pileggi C, Papadopoli R, Bianco A, Pavia M. Hepatitis B vaccine and the need for a booster dose after primary vaccination. Vaccine. 2017. DOI: 10.1016/j.vaccine.2017.09.076

[38] Bruce MG, Bruden D, Hurlburt D, Zanis C, Thompson G, Rea L, et al. Antibody levels and protection after Hepatitis B vaccine: Results of a 30-year follow-up study and response to a booster dose. The Journal of Infectious Diseases. 2016. DOI: 10.1093/infdis/jiv748

[39] Pybus OG, Barnes E, Taggart R, Lemey P, Markov PV, Rasachak B, et al. Genetic history of hepatitis C virus in East Asia. Journal of Virology. 2009;**83**:1071-1082. DOI: 10.1128/JVI.01501-08

[40] Choo QL, Kuo G, Weiner a J, Overby LR, Bradley DW, Houghton M. Isolation of a cDNA clone derived from a blood-borne non-A, non-B viral hepatitis genome. Science. 1989;**244**:359-362

[41] Lehman EM, Wilson ML. Epidemiology of hepatitis viruses among hepatocellular carcinoma cases and healthy people in Egypt: A systematic review and meta-analysis. International Journal of Cancer. 2009;**124**:690-697. DOI: 10.1002/ijc.23937

[42] Beaumont E, Roch E, Chopin L, Roingeard P. Hepatitis C virus E1 and E2 proteins used as separate immunogens induce neutralizing antibodies with additive properties. PLoS One. 2016. DOI: 10.1371/journal.pone.0151626

[43] Chevaliez S, Pawlotsky J-M. HCV genome and life cycle. In: Tan S-L, editor. Hepatitis C Viruses: Genomes and Molecular Biology. Norfolk, UK: Horizon Bioscience; 2006. pp. 5-48. PMID: 21250393

[44] Baumert TF, Ito S, Wong DT, Liang TJ. Hepatitis C virus structural proteins assemble into viruslike particles in insect cells. Journal of Virology. 1998;**72**:3827-3836

[45] Khan AG, Whidby J, Miller MT, Scarborough H, Zatorski AV, Cygan A, et al. Structure of the core ectodomain of the hepatitis C virus envelope glycoprotein 2. Nature. 2014. DOI: 10.1038/nature13117

[46] Fukuhara T, Ono C, Puig-Basagoiti F, Matsuura Y. Roles of lipoproteins and apolipoproteins in particle formation of Hepatitis C virus. Trends in Microbiology. 2015. DOI: 10.1016/j.tim.2015.07.007

[47] Yamamoto S, Fukuhara T, Ono C, Uemura K, Kawachi Y, Shiokawa M, et al. Lipoprotein receptors redundantly participate in entry of Hepatitis C virus. PLoS Pathogens. 2016. DOI: 10.1371/journal.ppat.1005610

[48] Diaz O, Delers F, Maynard M, Demignot S, Zoulim F, Chambaz J, et al. Preferential association of Hepatitis C virus with apolipoprotein B48-containing lipoproteins. The Journal of General Virology. 2006;**87**:2983-2991. DOI: 10.1099/vir.0.82033-0

[49] Felmlee DJ, Sheridan DA, Bridge SH, Nielsen SU, Milne RW, Packard CJ, et al. Intravascular transfer contributes to postprandial increase in numbers of very-low-density hepatitis C virus particles. Gastroenterology. 2010;**139**:1774-1783, 1783.e1-6. DOI: 10.1053/j.gastro.2010.07.047

[50] Kong L, Giang E, Nieusma T, Kadam RU, Cogburn KE, Hua Y, et al. Hepatitis C virus E2 envelope glycoprotein core structure. Science. 2013. DOI: 10.1126/science.1243876

[51] Dao Thi VL, Dreux M, Cosset F-L. Scavenger receptor class B type I and the hypervariable region-1 of hepatitis C virus in cell entry and neutralisation. Expert Reviews in Molecular Medicine. 2011;**13**:e13. DOI: 10.1017/S1462399411001785

[52] Boyer A, Dumans A, Beaumont E, Etienne L, Roingeard P, Meunier J-C. The association of hepatitis C virus glycoproteins with apolipoproteins E and B early in assembly is conserved in lipoviral particles. The Journal of Biological Chemistry. 2014;**289**:18904-18913. DOI: 10.1074/jbc.M113.538256

[53] Shawa IT, Sheridan DA, Felmlee DJ, Cramp ME. Lipid interactions influence hepatitis C virus susceptibility and resistance to infection. Clinics in Liver Disease. 2017;**10**:17-20. DOI: 10.1002/cld.643

[54] Sheridan DA, Hajarizadeh B, Fenwick FI, Matthews GV, Applegate T, Douglas M, et al. Maximum levels of hepatitis C virus lipoviral particles are associated with early and persistent infection. Liver International. 2016;**23**. DOI: 10.1111/liv.13176

[55] Barth H, Schafer C, Adah MI, Zhang F, Linhardt RJ, Toyoda H, et al. Cellular binding of hepatitis C virus envelope glycoprotein E2 requires cell surface heparan sulfate. The Journal of Biological Chemistry. 2003;**278**:41003-41012. DOI: 10.1074/jbc.M302267200

[56] Ramasamy I. Recent advances in physiological lipoprotein metabolism. Clinical Chemistry and Laboratory Medicine. 2014;**52**:1695-1727. DOI: 10.1515/cclm-2013-0358

[57] Filipe A, McLauchlan J. Hepatitis C virus and lipid droplets: Finding a niche. Trends in Molecular Medicine. 2015;**21**:34-42. DOI: 10.1016/j.molmed.2014.11.003

[58] Bassendine MF, Sheridan DA, Bridge SH, Felmlee DJ, Neely RDG. Lipids and HCV. Seminars in Immunopathology. 2013;**35**:87-100. DOI: 10.1007/s00281-012-0356-2

[59] Mysore KR, Leung DH. Hepatitis B and C. Clinics in Liver Disease. 2018. DOI: 10.1016/j.cld.2018.06.002

[60] Nelson PK, Mathers BM, Cowie B, Hagan H, Des Jarlais D, Horyniak D, et al. Global epidemiology of hepatitis B and hepatitis C in people who inject drugs: Results of systematic reviews. Lancet. 2011;**378**:571-583. DOI: 10.1016/S0140-6736(11)61097-0

[61] Bukh J. The history of hepatitis C virus (HCV): Basic research reveals unique features in phylogeny, evolution and the viral life cycle with new perspectives for epidemic control. Journal of Hepatology. 2016;**65**:S2-S21. DOI: 10.1016/j.jhep.2016.07.035

[62] Messina JP, Humphreys I, Flaxman A, Brown A, Cooke GS, Pybus OG, et al. Global distribution and prevalence of

hepatitis C virus genotypes. Hepatology. 2015;**61**:77-87. DOI: 10.1002/hep.27259

[63] Esteban JI, Sauleda S, Quer J. The changing epidemiology of hepatitis C virus infection in Europe. Journal of Hepatology. 2008;**48**:148-162. DOI: 10.1016/j.jhep.2007.07.033

[64] Bunchorntavakul C, Chavalitdhamrong D, Tanwandee T. Hepatitis c genotype 6: A concise review and response-guided therapy proposal. World Journal of Hepatology. 2013;**5**:496-504. DOI: 10.4254/wjh.v5.i9.496

[65] Thong VD, Akkarathamrongsin S, Poovorawan K, Tangkijvanich P, Poovorawan Y. Hepatitis C virus genotype 6: Virology, epidemiology, genetic variation and clinical implication. World Journal of Gastroenterology. 2014;**20**:2927-2940. DOI: 10.3748/wjg.v20.i11.2927

[66] Murphy DG, Sablon E, Chamberland J, Fournier E, Dandavino R, Tremblay CL. Hepatitis C virus genotype 7, a new genotype originating from Central Africa. Journal of Clinical Microbiology. 2015;**53**:967-972. DOI: 10.1128/JCM.02831-14

[67] Petruzziello A, Marigliano S, Loquercio G, Cozzolino A, Cacciapuoti C. Global epidemiology of hepatitis C virus infection: An up-date of the distribution and circulation of hepatitis C virus genotypes. World Journal of Gastroenterology. 2016;**22**:7824-7840. DOI: 10.3748/wjg.v22.i34.7824

[68] Williams JL, Cagle HH, Christensen CJ, Fox-Leyva LK, McMahon BJ. Results of a hepatitis C general transfusion lookback program for patients who received blood products before July 1992. Transfusion. 2005;**45**:1020-1026. DOI: 10.1111/j.1537-2995.2005.04280.x

[69] Gibb DM, Goodall RL, Dunn DT, Healy M, Neave P, Cafferkey M, et al. Mother-to-child transmission of hepatitis C virus: Evidence for preventable peripartum transmission. Lancet. 2000;**356**:904-907. DOI: 10.1097/00006454-200106000-00025

[70] Shawa IT, Felmlee DJ, Hegazy D, Sheridan DA, Cramp ME. Exploration of potential mechanisms of HCV resistance in exposed uninfected intravenous drug users. Journal of Viral Hepatitis. 2017;**24**(12):1082-1088. DOI: 10.1111/jvh.12720

[71] Thurairajah PH, Hegazy D, Chokshi S, Shaw S, Demaine A, Kaminski ER, et al. Hepatitis C virus (HCV)—Specific T cell responses in injection drug users with apparent resistance to HCV infection. The Journal of Infectious Diseases. 2008;**198**:1749-1755. DOI: 10.1086/593337

[72] Mizukoshi E, Eisenbach C, Edlin BR, Newton KP, Raghuraman S, Weiler-Normann C, et al. Hepatitis C virus (HCV)-specific immune responses of long-term injection drug users frequently exposed to HCV. The Journal of Infectious Diseases. 2008;**198**:203-212. DOI: 10.1086/589510

[73] Ghany MG, Jake Liang T. Natural history of chronic hepatitis C. In: Miyamura T, Lemon S, Walker C, Wakita T, editors. Hepatitis C Virus II: Infection and Disease. Tokyo, Japan: Springer; 2016. DOI: 10.1007/978-4-431-56101-9_1

[74] Hoshida Y, Fuchs BC, Bardeesy N, Baumert TF, Chung RT. Pathogenesis and prevention of hepatitis C virus-induced hepatocellular carcinoma. Journal of Hepatology. 2014;**61**:S79-S90. DOI: 10.1016/j.jhep.2014.07.010

[75] Esteban-Riesco L, Depaulis F, Moreau A, Bacq Y, Dubois F, Goudeau A, et al. Rapid and sustained autologous neutralizing response leading to early spontaneous recovery after HCV

infection. Virology. 2013;**444**:90-99. DOI: 10.1016/j.virol.2013.05.037

[76] Bunchorntavakul C, Jones LM, Kikuchi M, Reddy KR, Chang K. Distinct features in natural history and outcomes of acute Hepatitis C. Journal of Clinical Gastroenterology. 2015;**49**(4):e31-e40

[77] Li HC, Lo SY. Hepatitis C virus: Virology, diagnosis and treatment. World Journal of Hepatology. 2015;**7**:1377-1389. DOI: 10.4254/wjh.v7.i10.1377

[78] De Monte A, Courjon J, Anty R, Cua E, Naqvi A, Mondain V, et al. Direct-acting antiviral treatment in adults infected with hepatitis C virus: Reactivation of hepatitis B virus coinfection as a further challenge. Journal of Clinical Virology. 2016;**78**:27-30. DOI: 10.1016/j.jcv.2016.02.026

[79] Kondili LA, Robbins S, Blach S, Gamkrelidze I, Zignego AL, Brunetto MR, et al. Forecasting Hepatitis C liver disease burden on real-life data. Does the hidden iceberg matter to reach the elimination goals? Liver International. 2018;**38**:2190-2198. DOI: 10.1111/liv.13901

Chapter 5

Challenges and Strategies for Access to Treatment of Hepatitis C in Latin America

David Kershenobich and Nayelli Flores

Abstract

With the advent of all oral direct-acting antiviral drugs (DAAs) with a low incidence of side effects and very high success rates, we are entering an exciting new era in the treatment of hepatitis C virus (HCV), and now the major goal is the elimination of this viral infection. However, at least in Latin America, there are multiple barriers that must be attended.

Keywords: hepatitis C, direct-acting antiviral, treatment access, virus elimination, public health

1. Introduction

We are witnessing a new era in the treatment of HCV infection due to the development of DAAs that allows to cure a chronic disease without an effective vaccine. The therapy with pegylated interferon and ribavirin is no longer the standard of care. Unfortunately, there is a gap between these advances and the real access to treatment for patients in low- and middle-income countries (LMIC). In Latin America, the main identified barrier to access to hepatitis C treatment was for long a time the high price of these DAAs. While this issue has not yet been fully resolved, it has become evident that there are other gaps that need to be attended in order to undertake a comprehensive viral hepatitis elimination effort [1]. In this chapter, we propose to portray the main challenges that have not allowed fulfilling this purpose and present new strategies that could contribute toward addressing this health challenge.

2. Challenges to effectively treat HCV infection in Latin America

Chronic HCV infection is a health problem that affects more than 71 million people worldwide. HCV is associated with several hepatic pathologies, including cirrhosis and hepatocellular carcinoma as well as many other extrahepatic manifestations that are a major cause of global health burden [2].

The real incidence of hepatitis C and cirrhosis in Latin America is unknown. It has been estimated that at least 10 million Latin Americans may be infected with HCV [3, 4]. In some Latin American countries that provided national data, cirrhosis death rates were between 5 and 17/100,000 for men and 3 and 5/100,000 for women [5].

Liver cirrhosis mortality trends vary widely among countries in Latin America. Mortality rates increased in Costa Rica, Guatemala, Honduras, and Paraguay, but fell in Chile, Mexico, and Argentina. In 1980, age-standardized cirrhosis mortality rates in Chile and Mexico were, respectively, 53.4 (43.6–67.9) per 100,000 and 45.9 (35.6–57.0) per 100,000, the highest in the region. In 2010, Mexico remained the country with the highest cirrhosis mortality rate in the region, at 38.3 (30.7–47.5) per 100,000. Liver cirrhosis was the fourth leading cause of death in Mexico in 2010, accounting for 18% of deaths in males aged 40–49 years [6]. Disability, quality of life, and social aspects should be considered when assessing the impact of the disease.

2.1 Lack of epidemiological studies

Overall updated population-based epidemiological studies of viral hepatitis in most Latin American countries are still a significant challenge. This barrier is crucial to define health policies in the region [7]. There is a paucity of epidemiological data from rural areas where a significant percentage of the population resides. Most data are focused on seroprevalence of the disease, and studies are typically cross-sectional in design. Most of the studies have been conducted in select populations and do not allow to gain the real prevalence and incidence of HCV infection.

Efforts have been made to model the disease in some countries of the region, such as Mexico, Brazil, Argentina, and Chile. All of them indicate that if the number of patients identified and treated do not increase over the years, HCV-related morbidity and mortality are expected to increase, and the impact on the development of liver cirrhosis and hepatocarcinoma may be overwhelming [8].

In Mexico, for example, with the majority of cases arising from transfusion prior to the implementation of blood screening protocol, the annual number of HCV infection was estimated to peak in the mid-1990s. The annual number of new cases was estimated at 5620 new cases in 2013 [9].

In 2013, the total number of viremic infections was estimated at 560,700 (326, 900–605,200), and it was forecasted to decrease to 406,100 viremic infections in 2030. The number of HCC cases in 2013 was estimated at 2660 cases, and it was forecasted to increase by 55% by 2030. The number of liver-related deaths will increase by 55% from a base of 2370, while decompensated cirrhosis and compensated cirrhosis infections will increase 55 and 40% from a base of 6750 and 54,460 in 2013 [9].

In Argentina, there were an estimated 342,300 (155,000–537,000) infected individuals in 2013. Prevalence is estimated to have peaked at 382,700 patients in 2002 and to decline to 237,000 by 2030. There will be 62,630 compensated cirrhotic patients in 2030 as compared to 37,110 in 2013. In addition, there will be 3510 cases of HCC, and 8470 patients will be progressing to decompensated cirrhosis by 2030. Liver-related deaths in 2030 will number 3060 as compared to 1550 deaths in 2013. In 2013, 13% of viremic cases are estimated to have compensated cirrhosis or more advanced liver disease (decompensated cirrhosis, HCC, or transplant), while this proportion will increase to 32% in 2030 [9].

This type of epidemiological pattern is most likely to occur in the different countries through Latin America unless diagnostic and treatment rates of the HCV infection are increased.

2.2 Inadequate awareness and screening

Worldwide, the number of people that are aware of the diagnosis of hepatitis C is low. One of the challenges with diagnosing HCV infection is that it is often asymptomatic and that individuals seek medical attention only when they develop symptoms or signs of liver disease. In Mexico, for example, the average age at diagnosis of hepatitis C is 60.7 years, and 44% of them have liver cirrhosis, indicating that patients are arriving late for diagnosis and treatment [10–12].

Screening for HCV infection is central for identifying unknown cases. The early diagnosis of HCV infection can help to reduce the burden of disease and limit transmission to those at risk of infection or reinfection. Screening is critical to achieving the WHO targets by 2030 [13].

A high percentage of HCV-infected people lives in countries with limited resources to screen and treat hepatitis C. Latin America needs to overcome numerous challenges such as the lack of awareness among health professionals and the public in general. Each country in the region needs to plan its public health policy and screening strategy, but overall linkage to care remains an important hurdle.

2.3 Political disinterest

Political interest around the issue of hepatitis C treatment is uneven in the Latin American region. While affordability of DAAs has improved significantly in some countries such as Brazil, Mexico, Colombia, and Argentina, through strategies such as facilitating and speeding up the registration of the new DAAs, negotiating prices, compulsory licensing or generic competition, and exploring financial means by governments, insurance companies, or patients remain a significant task to undertake [14].

Access to treatment in different countries of Latin America is not systematic as they organize their healthcare in diverse ways so that eligibility and availability criteria vary significantly. Furthermore, specific guidance about health care entitlement is either not available, unclear, or not followed by medical professionals involved in diagnosing and treating hepatitis C.

2.4 Insufficient health care providers

Another important barrier restricting access to treatment in Latin America, particularly for the inhabitants with the lowest resources, is the limitations of providers of care. As a result, the number of patients referred for subspecialist evaluation remains low, and even when it occurs, patients may face long-distance travel, extended waiting time, and a lack of scheduling flexibility [15].

Among primary care provider's risk factors for HCV infection are not regularly sought, and deficiencies in HCV testing represent an additional barrier. Knowledge of HCV is generally inadequate.

Limited liver specialist availability through the region further contributes to the restriction of widespread opportunity of receiving treatment.

2.5 Identification of new risk factors

Risk factors for hepatitis C have changed over the years. A lack of knowledge regarding risk factors and treatment may contribute to low cure rates [16]. As blood bank screening has become almost universal, prevention and control of HCV should focus on recognizing high-risk population. In addition, rural populations, especially in areas with lower economic provision, should be under more attention. Evidence reported that intravenous or intranasal drug use and incarceration as well as the presence of hepatitis C in special populations such as patients with chronic renal failure in pre-dialysis, those in hemodialysis or co-infected individuals with HIV/hepatitis B are independent indicators of risk for past or present HCV infection [17]. The evolution of these risk factors will provide insights into understanding the future burden of hepatitis C.

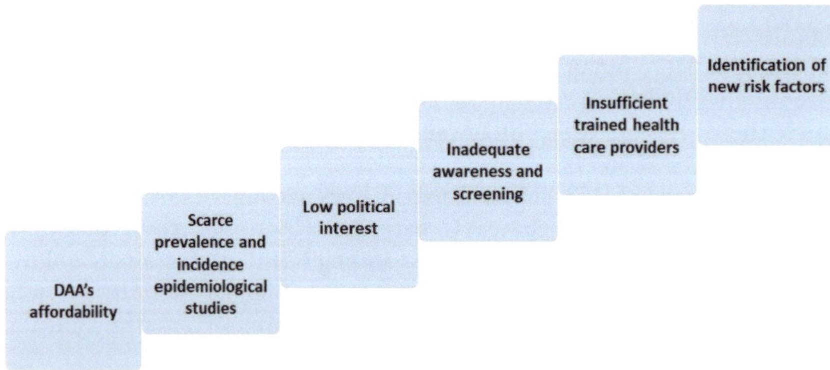

Figure 1.
Challenges to effectively treat HCV infection in Latin America.

Another important issue is the recognition that people remain at risk of reinfection with hepatitis C virus (HCV), even after clearance of the primary infection [18]. A significant issue is the recognition of cofactors that can accelerate progression of hepatic fibrosis in patients with HCV, such as obesity, diabetes mellitus, co-infection with HIV or hepatitis B, and alcohol consumption [19].

In order to achieve the continuum of care, identification of challenges in the region becomes very important. Special attention must be given at individual countries as their challenges may differ in their impact and significance (**Figure 1**).

3. Strategies for accessing HCV infection treatment

3.1 Conducting national campaigns of information and detection of hepatitis C in the general population

A social communication strategy is required to increase the perception that hepatitis C is a preventable and curable disease. It is necessary to educate the population about the risk factors and easy access to screening, utilizing massive ways of communication such as newspaper, magazine, book publishing, as well as radio, television, internet, film, and social media. It is important to make sure that messages are backed up by data in order to avoid confusion and being visionary to provide a good reason to attend the message. The inclusion of the rapid test should be recommended as part of routine test in medical examinations of high-risk individuals. This test allows point-of-care testing that can take place outside the clinical laboratory and can be administered and interpreted by nonspecialists, the results are available in 5–10 min, and its sensibility is 95–99% and specificity 99–100% [20]. In those cases with a positive test, it is necessary to determine a viral load to detect viremic cases and guarantee access to treatment.

3.2 Training programs for medical and nursing staff

It is recommendable to expand the number of health care professionals who can diagnose and administer DAAs, especially in rural areas fostering engagement in the continuum of care. Primary care physicians are in an ideal position to offer screening and diagnosis. Patients with advanced liver disease or complicated cases should be referred to the gastroenterologist, infectious disease specialist, or hepatologist. Nurses are at the forefront of providing information about the spread and diagnosis and treatment options available [21].

To pursue this goal, we propose to connect health teams from remote areas with specialists in medical centers in order to promote the continuity of patient care.

The training course includes:

- Epidemiology of HCV infection.
- Transmission of HCV infection.
- Detection of HCV infection in risk groups.
- Treatment of HCV infection.
- Strategies for the prevention of hepatitis C.

The Extension for Community Healthcare Outcomes (ECHO) model by the University of New Mexico Health Sciences Center (UNMHSC) has developed a platform to deliver complex specialty medical care to underserved populations through an innovative educational model of team-based interdisciplinary development. Using state-of-the-art telehealth technology, best practice protocols, and case-based learning, ECHO trains and supports primary care providers to develop knowledge and self-efficacy in hepatitis. ECHO has signed agreements in some Latin American countries which will contribute to advance the continuum of care for hepatitis C [22].

These types of programs will increase the familiarization of hepatitis C among general practitioners and nurses. They can be implemented taking advantage of the structure of the available health subsystems in every Latin American country.

3.3 Implementation of central laboratories to perform diagnostic tests

Rural communities face barriers when accessing health services, including facilities to perform laboratory studies. Latin America is confirmed by a diverse group of countries with great urban and rural disparities. Their health systems are usually structured in three levels: national, state, and local or their equivalents for every nation. Since 1990 every country in the region has gone through a series of health sector reforms with the aim of increasing equity, effectiveness, and coverage of health systems; unfortunately, despite their positive results, they have not achieved the proposed goals.

An important strategy would be the implementation of point-of-care testing in rural areas and instrument the structure to send blood samples to central laboratories when necessary. One of the primary goals of central laboratories is to achieve a 48-hour or less turnaround on the shipment of laboratory specimens from laboratory sites to the central lab location. These laboratories must have minimum levels of infrastructure, human resources, and quality standards to guarantee technical competence in the analytical framework. At the local level, this reference network could be established at health centers, hospitals, or other places defined by the state, with operational scope within a geographical area.

3.4 Regional programs to integrate medical specialists and health care providers from the prisons and addiction centers

Among these populations prevalence of hepatitis C is markedly increased and has been documented between 4 and 96% in several studies [23]. They are by far undiagnosed and unlinked to care. Very seldom do they seek medical attention unless they present overt clinical liver disease. As a preventive strategy, these patients should be screened actively, diagnosed, and be treated with DAAs. Treatment programs should include opiate substitution treatment and various harm reduction programs, including needle exchange programs. Ideally, these services should be delivered in the same place with an integrated approach [24, 25].

In the annual budgets of the prisons, it is necessary to foresee human and material resources to ensure they have medical facilities that improve HCV screening by point-of-care testing, outreach methods with mobile teams, rapid tests, and FibroScan to allow them to offer access to DAAs. We must strengthen the system of general prevention of hepatitis among all inmates as well.

3.5 Providing care in hospitals with focus on high-risk populations

A micro-elimination strategy should be implemented at individual hospitals, screening, diagnosing, and treating high-risk population attending for medical care. These populations include patients with liver diseases, patients with chronic renal failure, patients in pre-dialysis, patients with solid organ transplants, hemophiliacs, diabetics, and immunosuppressed patients from different etiologies as well as those pursuing emergency care. The micro-elimination strategy at these places should include the medical and paramedical personnel.

At the level of hospitals and health centers, an anonymous record of information on patients with hepatitis C should be implemented. This registry will provide epidemiological information on the route of acquisition of the disease, comorbidities and barriers to treatment access and document the response to DAAs and serve as an instrument that permits recording follow-up.

3.6 Simplification of bureaucratic procedures

Often in Latin American countries, access to DAAs is mired in bureaucracy implying excessive requirements difficult to meet for both patient and doctors. It is necessary to speed up the process in order to reduce the long queue of medication assignment, awaiting approval response, and shorten the long queue of medications awaiting review. At the institutional level, the form of payment (refund) of the medication can take months or years, so this is another important issue to overcome in order to make DAAs easily accessible.

Higher rates of DAA treatment must be accompanied by efficient screening, increased awareness, and more prescribers. It is necessary to innovate in the screening process, uncovering previously unidentified cases and those in the greatest need of treatment or at a high risk of transmitting the infection.

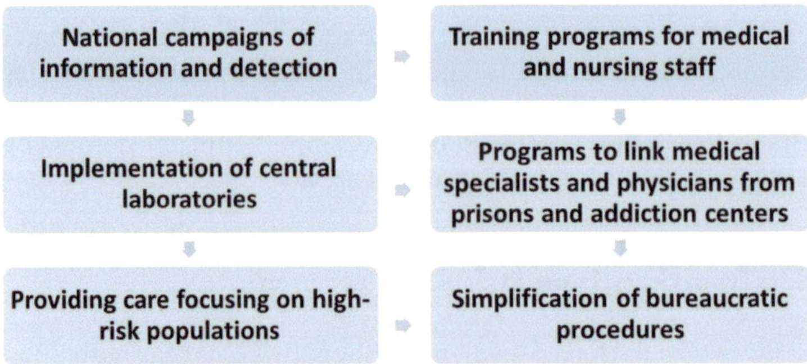

Figure 2.
Strategies for accessing HCV infection treatment.

Understanding the care cascade is vital for eliminating the virus. Reducing the HCV burden requires educational effort and scale-up of DAA therapies. The simplicity of oral regimens that are effective across HCV genotypes expands the number of physicians that can prescribe DAAs with scalable treatment models. Novel prescription systems are being developed, whereby internists and general practitioners may be eligible to prescribe DAAs in consultation with specialists (**Figure 2**).

4. Conclusions

Hepatitis C in Latin America has now become an important health issue. Strategies to identify patients have changed over time, shifting from blood bank to occult patients in high-risk populations (**Figure 3**). Implementation of treatment access is the main objective in order to achieve the WHO strategy of elimination by 2030. The pathway toward this goal is flagged by several barriers, including simplified detection, drug costs, public and professional education, awareness, and government concern, so the majority of HCV-infected individuals can benefit from the new generation of HCV antivirals.

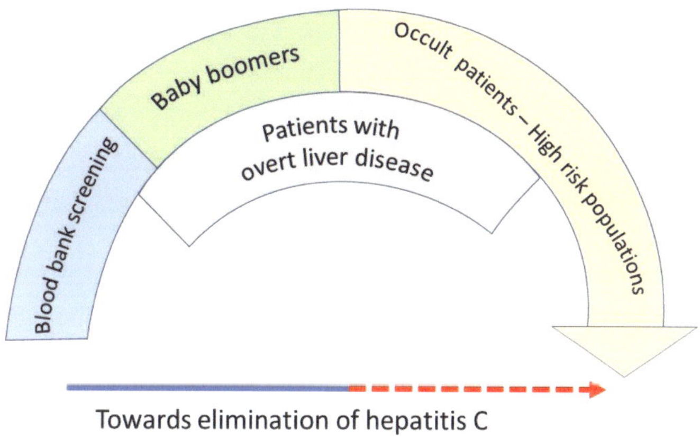

Figure 3.
Hepatitis C a Global Health issue.

Strategies to eliminate HCV infection must emphasize that this is a curable and preventable disease. As therapeutic regimens have become simpler and almost without side effects, the number of health care professionals who can diagnose and administer hepatitis C treatment is expanding the number of patients accessing treatment.

Conflict of interest

The authors declare no conflict of interest.

Author details

David Kershenobich* and Nayelli Flores
National Institute of Medical Sciences and Nutrition Salvador Zubirán,
Mexico City, Mexico

*Address all correspondence to: kesdhipa@yahoo.com

References

[1] Graham CS, Swan T. A path to eradication of hepatitis C in low-and middle-income countries. Antiviral Research. 2015;**119**:89-96. DOI: 10.1016/j.antiviral.2015.01.004

[2] Thrift AP, El-Serag HB, Kanwal F. Global epidemiology and burden of HCV infection and HCV-related disease. Nature Reviews Gastroenterology and Hepatology. 2017;**14**:122-132. DOI: 10.1038/nrgastro.2016.176

[3] Chen DS, Hamoudi W, Mustapha B, Layden J, Nersesov A, Reic T, et al. Strategies to manage hepatitis C virus infection disease burden-Volume 4. Journal of Viral Hepatitis. 2017;**24**(Suppl 2):44-63. DOI: 10.1111/jvh.12759

[4] Panduro A, Roman S. Need of righteous attitudes toward eradication of hepatitis C virus infection in Latin America. World Journal of Gastroenterology. 2016;**22**:5137-5142. DOI: 10.3748/wjg.v22.i22.5137

[5] Davalos Moscol M, Bustos Sanchez C. The burden of hepatic encephalopathy in Latin America. Annals of Hepatology. 2011;(Suppl 2):31-35

[6] Mokdad AA, Lopez AD, Shahraz S, Lozano R, Mokdad AH, Stanaway K, et al. Liver cirrhosis mortality in 187 countries between 1980 and 2010: A systematic analysis. BMC Medicine. 2014;**12**:145. DOI: 10.1186/s12916-014-0145-y

[7] Botero RC, Tagle M. New therapies for hepatitis C: Latin American perspectives. Clinical Liver Disease. 2015;**5**:8-10. DOI: 10.1002/cld.438

[8] Gane E, Kershenobich D, Seguin-Devaux C, Kristian P, Aho I, Dalgard O, et al. Strategies to manage hepatitis C virus (HCV) infection disease burden–Volume 2. Journal of Viral Hepatitis. 2015;**22**(Suppl 1):46-73. DOI: 10.1111/jvh.12352

[9] Hatzakis A, Chulanov V, Gadano AC, Bergin C, Ben-Ari Z, Mossong J, et al. The present and future disease burden of hepatitis C virus (HCV) infections with today's treatment paradigm–Volume 2. Journal of Viral Hepatitis. 2015;**22**(Suppl 1):26-45. DOI: 10.1111/jvh.12351

[10] Corona-Lau C, Muñoz L, Wolpert E, Aguilar LM, Dehesa M, Gutiérrez C, et al. Hepatitis C screening in the general population. Revista de Investigación Clínica. 2015;**67**:104-108

[11] Lau-Corona D, Pineda LA, Avilés HH, Gutiérrez-Reyes G, Farfan-Labonne BE, Núñez-Nateras R, et al. Effective use of FibroTest to generate decision trees in hepatitis C. World Journal of Gastroenterology. 2009;**15**(21):2617-2622. DOI: 10.3748/wjg.15.2617

[12] Chirino RA, Dehesa M, Wolpert E, Corona-Lau C, García Juárez I, Sánchez Avila JF, et al. Chronic hepatitis C treatment with direct antiviral agents in a real-life setting. Revista de Investigación Clínica. 2016;**68**(4):203-212

[13] Shehata N, Austin T, Ha S, Timmerman K. Barriers to and facilitators of hepatitis C virus screening and testing: A scoping review. Canada Communicable Disease Report. 2018;**44**:166-172. DOI: 10.14745/ccdr.v44i78a03

[14] Kershenobich D, Torre A, Heading toward the elimination of Hepatitis C virus. Valenzuela LM. Revista de Investigación Clínica. 2018;**70**:29-31. DOI: 10.24875/RIC.18002467k

[15] Naffah F. Patients with hepatitis C are best managed by a specialist in

liver diseases. CON: The management of hepatitis C in a community-based practice. The American Journal of Gastroenterology. 2007;**102**:1839-1841. DOI: 10.1111/j.1572-0241.2007.01433_3.x

[16] Knick T, Sherbuk JE, Dillingham R. Knowledge of hepatitis C risk factors is lower in high incidence regions. The Journal of Community Health. 2018. DOI: 10.1007/s10900-018-0545-6. [Epub ahead of print]

[17] Bernieh B. Viral hepatitis in hemodialysis: An update. Journal of Translational Internal Medicine. 2015;**3**:93-105

[18] Young J, Rossi C, Gill J, Walmsley S, Cooper C, Cox J, et al. Risk factors for hepatitis C virus reinfection after sustained virologic response in patients coinfected with HIV. Clinical Infectious Diseases. 2017;**64**:1154-1162. DOI: 10.1093/cid/cix126

[19] Elpek GÖ. Cellular and molecular mechanisms in the pathogenesis of liver fibrosis: An update. World Journal of Gastroenterology. 2014;**20**:7260-7276. DOI: 10.3748/wjg.v20.i23.7260

[20] Tang W, Chen W, Amini A, Boeras D, Falconer J, Kelly H, et al. Diagnostic accuracy of tests to detect Hepatitis C antibody: A meta-analysis and review of the literature. Infectious Diseases. 2017;**17**(Suppl 1):695. DOI: 10.1186/s12879-017-2773-2

[21] Mellinger JL, Volk ML. Multidisciplinary management of patients with cirrhosis: A need for care coordination. Clinical Gastroenterology and Hepatology. 2013;**11**:217-223. DOI: 10.1016/j.cgh.2012.10.040

[22] Marciano S, Haddad L, Plazzotta F, Mauro E, Terraza S, Arora S, et al. Implementation of the ECHO® telementoring model for the treatment of patients with hepatitis C. Journal of Medical Virology. 2017;**89**:660-664. DOI: 10.1002/jmv.24668

[23] Degenhardt L, Peacock A, Colledge S, Leung J, Grebely J, Vickerman P, et al. Global prevalence of injecting drug use and sociodemographic characteristics and prevalence of HIV, HBV, and HCV in people who inject drugs: A multistage systematic review. Lancet Global Health. 2017;**5**:e1192-e1207. DOI: 10.1016/S2214-109X(17)30375-3

[24] Delile JM, de Ledinghen V, Jauffret-Roustide M, Roux P, Reiller B, Foucher J, et al. Hepatitis C virus prevention and care for drug injectors: The French approach. Hepatology, Medicine and Policy. 2018;**3**:7. DOI: 10.1186/s41124-018-0033-8

[25] Lemoine M, Thursz M. Hepatitis C, a global issue: Access to care and new therapeutic and preventive approaches in resource-constrained areas. Seminars in Liver Disease. 2014;**34**:89-97. DOI: 10.1055/s-0034-1371082

Chapter 6

Direct-Acting Antivirals in Chronic Hepatitis C Infection with Liver Cirrhosis

Vijay Gayam, Arshpal Gill, Pavani Garlapati and Smruti Mohanty

Abstract

Chronic hepatitis C infection is a common cause of liver morbidity and mortality across the world, in part due to complications including cirrhosis and hepatocellular carcinoma. The advent of Direct-acting antiviral (DAA) therapy has the potential to change the outcome of HCV infection in the vast majority of patients. Unfortunately, the chronic nature of HCV infection means that many patients requiring direct-acting antiviral (DAA) therapy have already developed compensated cirrhosis. This chapter reviews the importance of DAAs in the treatment of HCV infection, particularly in patients with existing compensated cirrhosis. Both efficacy and safety are discussed as essential endpoints of DAA therapy. Decompensated cirrhosis, treatment failures, vitamin-D deficiency, HIV co-infection, and ethnic differences in the context of treatment response are also discussed in this chapter.

Keywords: direct-acting antivirals, chronic hepatitis C, hepatitis C virus, liver cirrhosis, treatment, adverse drug events

1. Introduction

Hepatitis C virus (HCV) is a leading cause of virologic morbidity and mortality, and afflicted individuals with HCV remain at high risk of cirrhosis, hepatic failure, and hepatocellular carcinoma [1]. The dormant nature of the Hepatitis C virus enables the virus to be both transmissible and silent. This may result in a more advanced initial presentation, as many patients are unaware of their positive infection status [2]. More advanced stages of HCV may involve cirrhosis, one of the most morbid outcomes after initial infection with HCV infection. As a result, many patients requiring HCV therapy are already cirrhotic and require a therapy which can effectively combat HCV in both non-cirrhotic and cirrhotic stages of the disease. The importance of treating the HCV virus in the compensated cirrhosis stage is paramount, to prevent the enhanced risk of worsening cirrhosis, decompensation, hepatocellular carcinoma, and death [1].

The original treatment option in chronic HCV infection was interferon-based regimens. Interferon-based regimens were once the mainstay of therapy, but it has limited effectiveness in their ability to consistently induce a sustained virologic response (SVR) in chronic HCV at high enough rates to be a plausible solution for HCV [3]. Due to the infectious and chronic nature of hepatitis C, a more successful therapy than interferon-based therapy was warranted to reduce the global burden of disease. In addition to its ineffectiveness, interferon-based regimens had numerous side effects. The side effects are often severe and debilitating, which included bone marrow depression, neuropsychiatric symptoms, and flu-like symptoms. These side effects likely contributed to reduced patient adherence to interferon therapy [3].

The development of effective antiviral therapy for HCV infection was a difficult challenge. HCV exhibits some features which can make it difficult to treat. The HCV has a 9600-nucleotide positive sense RNA genome. The viral polymerase of HCV is unable to replicate at a high fidelity allowing for numerous errors. There is also a high viral replication rate. These two factors allow for the existence of diverse quasi-species, and in turn, the quasi-species makes both host immune response and pharmacological interventions less effective [2]. Fortunately, the new effective treatment was developed with the introduction of direct-acting antivirals (DAAs) for HCV infection. DAAs appear to meet the challenge of consistently inducing a high SVR in hepatitis C patients, including in patients who have already developed compensated cirrhosis.

2. The natural history of chronic hepatitis C and compensated cirrhosis

HCV is a blood-borne virus and will result in chronic infection in 55–85% of patients. Once the infection is chronic, patients are unlikely to have spontaneous resolution of their infection and are thus at risk of fibrosis, cirrhosis, and hepatocellular carcinoma. Approximately 20–30% of patients with chronic HCV infection will develop cirrhosis [1]. There are numerous host factors in determining whether or not there will be a chronic infection, including IL-28B polymorphisms which may be associated with spontaneous resolution of the infection [2]. The development of cirrhosis at a cellular level is due to the virus inducing CD8+ T cell inflammation and necrosis, which is then followed by eventual healing via fibro-genesis pathways. This cycle of insult and healing can result in cirrhosis after 10–20 years of viral hepatitis [4].

Cirrhosis is a significant cause of detriment in the chronic HCV infection and ultimately can lead to the end stages of HCV infection, including decompensation, hepatocellular carcinoma (HCC), death, or the need for transplantation [5]. Decompensated cirrhotic patients HCV develop encephalopathy, ascites, or variceal bleed. Both variceal hemorrhage and HCC represent the fatal consequences of chronic HCV and cirrhosis [5]. Numerous studies done on DAAs and prevention of hepatocellular carcinoma indicate that DAA therapy does ultimately decrease the overall risk of HCC [6–8]. However, even with DAA therapy there still may be an increased risk of HCC in patients with treated HCV infection, so the exact benefit of DAAs on the reduction of HCC in patients who have existing HCV infection is unknown [9, 10]. Due to the uncertainty of the exact benefit of DAAs on HCC, patients with HCV and compensated cirrhosis should undergo HCC screenings, including those who have already completed a DAA regimen and achieved SVR.

DAA therapy is a relatively new concept and was designed to directly inhibit the viral lifecycle. In addition to the antiviral benefit, there is early evidence to indicate that DAA therapy is concurrently reducing HCV-associated manifestations including cirrhosis and cirrhosis-related complications [6]. Evidence of DAA therapy's protective benefit from HCV cirrhosis-related complications can be seen in transplant databases. There is a relationship between DAA therapy and the decreased need for HCV-associated liver transplants [11]. This is of significant benefit, as a liver transplant represents the most expensive financial burden HCV can place on a healthcare system, and by being able to mitigate this expense, DAAs may not only prove to be effective therapeutically but also economically [12].

While one of the most important goals of treating HCV is to prevent cirrhosis; a significant portion of HCV patients already have existing cirrhosis in need of DAA therapy. Furthermore, these patients are more likely to have DAA treatment failure versus their non-cirrhotic counterparts [13]. This makes DAA therapy of paramount significance for clinicians, in both preventing HCV cirrhosis and emphasizing the importance of selecting an appropriate DAA regimen in HCV patients with compensated cirrhosis.

3. Direct-acting antiviral agents

DAAs were first approved by the Food and Drug Administration (FDA) in 2011 and were used initially with the old standard of care interferon-based regimens [14]. DAAs can be classified into four different groups; protease inhibitors, polymerase inhibitors, NS5B inhibitors, and NS5A inhibits [14]. The primary mechanism of DAAs is to directly inhibit the lifecycle replication of HCV virus. There are also specific methods of resistance that the HCV virus may develop, and it is essential to consider the possibility of resistance when starting HCV therapy [15].

There are numerous regimens available involving DAAs. The American Association for the Study of Liver disease (AASLD) have developed HCV guidelines to assist in selecting a particular DAA regimen based on variables including the genotype of HCV infection, treatment naïve status, existing compensated cirrhosis, decompensated cirrhosis, and co-infection with HIV (**Table 1**) [16]. DAA is typically 8 or 12 weeks depending on the indication given in the AASLD guidelines along with the regimen being given. Overall, SVR rates appear high with DAA regimens [13]. The benefits of DAAs can also be observed in histological

Genotype	Drug	Treatment duration (weeks)
Genotype 1	Elbasvir/Grazoprevir	12
	Glecaprevir/Pibrentasvir	12
	Ledipasvir/Sofosbuvir	12
	Sofosbuvir/Velpatasvir	12
Genotype 2	Glecaprevir/Pibrentasvir	12
	Sofosbuvir/Velpatasvir	12
Genotype 3	Glecaprevir/Pibrentasvir	12
	Sofosbuvir/Velpatasvir	12
Genotype 4	Elbasvir/Grazoprevir	12
	Glecaprevir/Pibrentasvir	12
	Ledipasvir/Sofosbuvir	12
	Sofosbuvir/Velpatasvir	12
Genotype 5/6	Glecaprevir/Pibrentasvir	12
	Ledipasvir/Sofosbuvir	12
	Sofosbuvir/Velpatasvir	12

Table 1.
DAA regimens for each HCV major genotype in the treatment of patients with compensated cirrhosis, according to current AASLD guidelines.

studies. Patients who have achieved remission with DAAs show a lessened degree of inflammation on tissue specimen examination. Interestingly, there is no decrease in fibrosis noted at a histological level [17].

Successful DAA therapy is defined as a sustained virologic remission at 12 weeks (SVR12) post-treatment in the infected patient. The success of DAA therapy has a lot of variables, which is addressed in the AASLD guidelines. Corroborating an appropriate regimen based on a specific genotype, the presence of existing cirrhosis, HIV co-infection, treatment naivety, and treatment failure is all addressed in the AASLD guidelines [16]. In addition to the factors addressed in the AASLD guidelines, there appear to be some genetic examples influencing SVR in DAA therapy, include IL-28B polymorphisms, low-density lipid receptor genetic variants, vitamin D receptor, and bile salt export pump polymorphisms [18].

4. DAAs in the role of combating HCV as a public health problem

DAAs in conjunction with appropriate global health strategies provides us with the possibility to diminish HCV as a public health problem [19]. Analytical data collected from a treat-all model indicate there is a cost-effective benefit to treating all HCV infected individuals with DAA regimens [20]. Urbanization is another crucial factor to consider as increased rates of urbanization may be associated with the risk of HCV [21]. Not all endemic areas with HCV are countries of means, so it remains necessary to consider the price of antiviral regimens and eliminate any economic barriers towards achieving comprehensive treatment response. One study analyzing the cost of HCV treatment stated the current DAA price point appears to be affordable to treat most populations at an extensive level, similar to HIV. The same study concluded that genotype testing remains a significant cost until a consistent pan-genotypic DAA regimen can be developed [22]. The current DAA regimens and guidelines are contingent on knowing the genotype being treated. This is because much of the existing data in the literature shows a particular regimen's treatment success rates as a function of the genotype being treated [16].

Public health programs should also be instituted alongside DAA therapy to help reduce the burden of HCV infection. In the United States, intravenous drug users are responsible for a new increase in HCV infections; before this rise, the incidence of HCV had been decreasing [1]. Being able to both reduce the rate of new infections while treat existing infections with DAA regimens would make the most logistical sense in reducing the global burden of disease associated with HCV. In addition to the benefit of lowering HCV infections, the advent of DAAs could also reduce the global incidence of HCC as both hepatitis B and C are prominent identifiable risks for the development of HCC globally [23].

5. Hepatitis C genotypes

There are six major genotypes of HCV virus. There is a geographical component in HCV genotypes, as different regions of the world have a varying rate of the six different HCV genotypes. The information about HCV genotyping is significant, as it helps dictate therapy. The current AASLD guidelines rely primarily on genotype when assisting clinicians to select a particular DAA regimen. The genotype also provides pre-treatment success probabilities when selecting a DAA regimen for the achievement of SVR in patients with existing compensated cirrhosis. One study noted that HCV Genotype 1 patient with cirrhosis tend to have high SVR regardless of their cirrhosis status, but Genotype 3 patients have a more diminished response and are therefore more difficult to treat in existing cirrhosis [24]. Ribavirin may be used as an adjunct with DAA regimens to help achieve SVR in patients with specific characteristics, including the genotype. Below are the major six genotypes of HCV, and the current AASLD guidelines for each one with an emphasis on the management with compensated cirrhosis.

5.1 Genotype 1

Genotype 1 infection is the most common genotype globally, and it is also the most common genotype seen in developed countries [25]. Community-based studies conducted in the United States are often reflective of Genotype 1 infections as it is the predominant subtype in the United States, and Genotype 1 infections demonstrate a high overall SVR with DAA including in patients with existing cirrhosis [26].

5.1.1 Elbasvir/Grazoprevir

The C-WORTHY trial included patients that were both non-cirrhotic and existing compensated cirrhosis, with both groups being treated with Elbasvir/Grazoprevir. The SVR reflected the success rate in both patients without cirrhosis and with compensated cirrhosis. The conclusion can be made that compensated cirrhosis is not a hindrance in the achievement of SVR in patients taking Elbasvir/Grazoprevir [27]. The AASLD guidelines indicate 12 weeks of Elbasvir/Grazoprevir treatment is warranted in HCV Genotype 1 infections in both non-cirrhotic patients and in patients who have compensated cirrhosis [16].

5.1.2 Glecaprevir/Pibrentasvir

The EXPEDITION-1 study examined patients with compensated cirrhosis across genotypes 1, 2, 4, 5, and 6. Only genotype 3 was not represented among the six major genotypes. All 5 of the genotypes showed a high overall treatment response, with the genotype 1 patients with cirrhosis showing an SVR of 100% [28].

The CERTAIN-1 studied Japanese patients with genotype 1 infections, and also documented an excellent treatment response. The SVR remained high in patients with compensated cirrhosis, with all 38 cirrhotic patients achieving SVR [29]. The current AASLD guidelines mandate that non-cirrhotic, treatment naïve patients taking Glecaprevir/Pibrentasvir require 8 weeks of therapy, but the duration of therapy extends to 12 weeks with the presence of compensated cirrhosis [16].

5.1.3 Ledipasvir/Sofosbuvir

The ION-1 study showed high SVR rates in all treatment naïve patients with genotype 1 infection. The effect of cirrhosis on efficacy was difficult to determine, but there was no negative effect on the safety profile [30]. Ledipasvir/Sofosbuvir is an 8-week therapy in non-cirrhotic, non-black, non-HIV positive patients, but the presence of compensated cirrhosis changes the guidelines therapy to 12 weeks [16].

5.1.4 Sofosbuvir/Velpatasvir

Sofosbuvir/Velpatasvir is a 12-week regimen regardless of cirrhosis status [16]. The ASTRAL-1 examined patients who received Sofosbuvir/Velpatasvir for 12 weeks across genotype 1, 2, 4, 5, 6 with genotype 3 not being represented. Across all 5 genotypes studied, there were 121 patients in ASTRAL-1 with compensated cirrhosis. All but 1 achieved SVR (120/121), indicating a high success rate [31]. This may also help support the idea that Sofosbuvir/Velpatasvir could potentially be a pan-genotypic drug in compensated cirrhosis, as 5 of the six major genotypes were in this study.

5.2 Genotype 2 infection

Genotype 2 infection is most commonly seen in East Asia [25]. There are currently 2 AASLD recommended therapies for treatment naive Genotype 2 infections [16].

5.2.1 Glecaprevir/Pibrentasvir

The EXPEDITION-1 trial examined genotype 2 patients, and similar to the genotype 1 patients, genotype 2 patients with compensated cirrhosis achieved SVR at a high rate of 100% with Glecaprevir/Pibrentasvir [28]. These findings were reproduced in the CERTAIN-1 trial in Japan, with all 18 genotype 2 patients with compensated cirrhosis achieving SVR without any adverse drug reactions [32].

5.2.2 Sofosbuvir/Velpatasvir

The Sofosbuvir/Velpatasvir regimen to combat genotype 2 infections was studied in the ASTRAL-1 and ASTRAL-2 studies. The results showed that Sofosbuvir/Velpatasvir was effective at achieving SVR in genotype 2 infections (99%) and that SVR rates were not affected by cirrhosis [31].

5.3 Genotype 3 infection

After Genotype 1 infections, Genotype 3 infections are the most common type of HCV worldwide. Genotype 3 remains the most predominant type of HCV infection in South Asia [25]. Genotype 3 infections are a particular challenge when it comes to compensated cirrhosis. It is the second most common infection, but it does not respond well to first generation sofosbuvir-based regimens in the presence of cirrhosis. The ALLY-3 trial, involving the daclatasvir/sofosbuvir showed a response rate of 96% in patients without any cirrhosis. However, among patients with existing compensated cirrhosis, the response rate plummeted to a mere 63% [33].

5.3.1 Glecaprevir/Pibrentasvir

The Surveyor II study showed that with 12 weeks of therapy, treatment response was observed in 98% of Genotype 3 treatment naïve patients who had compensated cirrhosis [34]. The AASLD guidelines call for an 8-week therapy in treatment naïve patients without cirrhosis, but the presence of cirrhosis extends the Glecaprevir/Pibrentasvir therapy to 12 weeks.

5.3.2 Sofosbuvir/Velpatasvir

The ASTRAL-3 study showed a high overall SVR for genotype 3 patients taking Sofosbuvir/Velpatasvir. However, there was a reduction in SVR from 97% in patients with no cirrhosis down to 91% in patients with cirrhosis [35]. Although there was a decrease in efficacy due to the presence of cirrhosis, it was a far less drastic decrease when comparing the outcomes in Genotype 3 treatment with Daclatasvir/Sofosbuvir in the presence of cirrhosis [33]. The standard of treatment is 12 weeks, regardless of cirrhosis status [16].

5.4 Genotype 4 infection

Genotype 4 infections are seen in Africa and the Middle East, with Egypt, in particular, shouldering a high rate of HCV genotype 4 infections [25]. The response rate in genotype 4 infections appears to be high in some real-world studies, regardless of cirrhosis status [36].

5.4.1 Elbasvir/Grazoprevir

The current AASLD guidelines recommend a 12-week therapy, regardless of whether or not there is existing cirrhosis.

5.4.2 Glecaprevir/Pibrentasvir

EXPEDITION-1 showed that Genotype 4 patients with compensated cirrhosis still had a high SVR [28]. The AASLD guidelines dictate an 8-week regimen in patients with no history of cirrhosis, but the Glecaprevir/Pibrentasvir regimen becomes 12 weeks within patients with compensated cirrhosis.

5.4.3 Ledipasvir/Sofosbuvir

One study examined the success rate of Ledipasvir/Sofosbuvir with Genotype 4 infection; with all patients achieving SVR regardless of any underlying fibrosis or cirrhosis [37].

5.4.4 Sofosbuvir/Ledipasvir

ASTRAL-1 showed all patients with Sofosbuvir/Ledipasvir and a Genotype 4 infection achieved SVR12 [31]. The population studied had both patients with compensated cirrhosis and without cirrhosis patients, but both groups had an SVR of 100%. The AASLD mandates a 12-week therapy as the recommended regimen regardless of cirrhosis status.

5.5 Genotype 5 and genotype 6 infection

The current AASLD guidelines have HCV genotype 5 and genotype 6 infections grouped, but they remain 2 distinct major genotypes of HCV infection. Genotype 5 represents the least commonly observed genotype of the major HCV genotypes and is most commonly seen in Sub-Saharan Africa and East Africa. Genotype 6 infections are most commonly seen in East Asia [25].

5.5.1 Glecaprevir/Pibrentasvir

The EXPEDITION-1 trial showed that patients with compensated cirrhosis and both genotype 5 and genotype 6 infection achieved remission at high rates [28].

5.5.2 Ledipasvir/Sofosbuvir

Genotype 5 compensated cirrhosis patients had studied in one trial had a lower response rate than their non-cirrhotic counterparts [38]. However, there was just one non-responder in each group, with 8/9 cirrhotic patients achieving SVR (89%) and 31/32 patients without cirrhosis achieving SVR (97%). Both non-responders had an IL-28B polymorphism.

5.5.3 Sofosbuvir/Velpatasvir

Overall SVR12 was observed in patients with Genotype 5 and Genotype 6 infections at rates of 97% and 100%, respectively in ASTRAL-1. Compensated cirrhosis was included in both groups of patients, and across all 5 genotypes (1, 2, 4, 5, 6) studied in ASTRAL-1, 120/121 (99%) of patients with compensated cirrhosis achieved SVR [31].

6. Decompensated cirrhosis and direct acting anti-viral therapy

Patients with cirrhosis are at risk of hepatic decompensation, which includes ascites, encephalopathy, spontaneous bacterial peritonitis and variceal bleed [1]. The development of any one of these features represents increase mortality, and decompensation represents an end stage of HCV infection, with patients having a 5-year survival rate of 51% [39]. Decompensation also remains an independent risk factor for the development of HCC [40].

Selecting an appropriate DAA therapy in patients with compensated cirrhosis is therefore important, as it may help to avoid the morbidity and mortality associated with decompensated cirrhosis. There are a few DAA regimens which show benefit in patients who have decompensated cirrhosis.

Before DAAs, interferon-based regimens were the only option, and in particular, when discussing the decompensated population, interferon-based regimens were both ineffective and poorly tolerated [41].

The ALLY-1 study looked at the effects of Daclatasvir/Sofosbuvir along with ribavirin on patients with advanced cirrhosis, including decompensated cirrhosis across 5 of the 6 major HCV genotypes, with genotype 5 being the only one not represented [42]. They noted a high treatment response with Child-Pugh A or B cirrhosis (93%), but once progression to Child-Pugh C cirrhosis occurred, the efficacy of Daclatasvir/Sofosbuvir was significantly diminished with a treatment response of 56%.

ASTRAL-4 also demonstrated a diminished response to DAAs in decompensated cirrhosis. Among patients who received Sofosbuvir/Velpatasvir alone, the SVR was 83%. The addition of ribavirin however improved the SVR to 94% [43].

The adjunct use of ribavirin therapy and extending the duration may also be indicated in the treatment of HCV with decompensation according to current AASLD guidelines. Insulin resistance and protein malnutrition are two associated risks with the development of decompensated cirrhosis, so clinicians should be aware and attempt to address these issues to prevent further worsening of HCV into decompensation [44].

7. Direct-acting antivirals in HCV/HIV co-infected patients and compensated cirrhosis

The Human Immunodeficiency Virus (HIV) and Hepatitis C (HCV) are both blood-borne infections which share common risk factors with regards to routes of transmission. Intravenous drug users may be at risk of both infections, and intravenous drug users represent the most common cause of new HCV infections [1]. Co-infection with HCV and HIV also appears to alter the host immune system, with strong evidence of decreased natural killer cells [45]. Clinicians also must exercise caution as there remains a possibility of drug-drug interaction, including hepatotoxicity between Highly Active-Antiretroviral Therapy (HAART) and DAA

[2]. This is a stark contrast from interferon-based regimens, which both struggled to consistently induce SVR and had numerous patient discontinuations due to adverse events [46]. Daclatasvir/Sofosbuvir appears to have a high success across genotypes 1–4 as observed in the ALLY-2 study; with the success of Daclatasvir/Sofosbuvir being possibly contingent on favorable pharmacokinetics when interacting with HAART in HIV treatment. The SVR rates remained high even in patients with compensated cirrhosis, with a reported SVR of 92% in co-infected and cirrhotic patients The SVR was low with 8 weeks of therapy, and to achieve SVR of 92% patients required 12 weeks of treatment [47]. Community-based literature involving reiterate the idea that there may be a slightly diminished response in the HCV/HIV co-infected cohort in real-world studies [48].

8. Direct-acting antivirals in substance abuse patients with pre-existing cirrhosis

Substance abuse is a noteworthy variable when discussing hepatitis C virus and cirrhosis. Intravenous drug use and contaminated needles are now the most common way in which new cases of hepatitis C are contracted [1]. As a result, it is important to target the most common cause of new infections to help reduce the spread of hepatitis C virus. The AASLD guidelines currently recommend annual testing for the HCV virus alongside counseling on measures to reduce HCV transmission [16].

9. Direct-acting antivirals in the African-American population

The African-American population is an important population when it comes to chronic hepatitis C infection, as they have an infection rate three times higher than the non-Hispanic White population [49]. Interferon-based treats were less effective in African-Americans than other groups, so there is some historical significance in finding a consistently effective treatment [50]. Fortunately, DAAs appears to be effective in the African-American population with response rates being high and treatment not having a significant variation with a history of compensated cirrhosis [51, 52]. Ethnicity is a factor seen in the AASLD guidelines; for instance, patients who would otherwise need 8 weeks of Ledipasvir/Sofosbuvir would require 12 weeks due to African-American ethnicity [16].

10. Association of vitamin D level and HCV treatment response

Vitamin D deficiency appears to be a marker of hepatic dysfunction in patients who have the chronic liver disease and may be predictive of decompensation and mortality [53]. Vitamin D also has some molecular implications in the development of HCV related HCC [54]. Vitamin D deficiency is also noted to be more likely in patients with cirrhosis versus non-cirrhotic counterparts; although the levels of pre-treatment vitamin D does not appear to significantly influence SVR [55].

11. Management of non-responders

The AASLD treats patients who have failed interferon-based therapy in the same group as DAA naïve patients. DAAs remain effective treatment in the vast majority of patients with compensated cirrhosis. However, there remains a portion of the hepatitis C patient population who do not respond to DAA therapy. These patients pose a unique challenge.

The POLARIS-1 and POLARIS-4 trials involve patients who have failed DAA regimens across 4 genotypes (genotype 1, 2, 3, 4) and were given Sofosbuvir/Velpatasvir/Voxilaprevir. POLARIS-1 had an SVR of 96% in patients taking for re-treatment, with a 99% success in patients with no cirrhosis and 93% in patients with compensated cirrhosis. POLARIS-4 had an SVR of 98% and did not differ based on cirrhosis status [56]. The regimen of Sofosbuvir/Velpatasvir/Voxilaprevir appears to be an effective therapy in DAA treatment failures.

12. Safety and tolerability of direct-acting antivirals

The development of DAAs not only improved the efficacy of HCV treatment but also enhanced the safety and tolerability of HCV therapy. The improved safety profile and increased tolerability can be observed in both patients with and without compensated cirrhosis. It is important to continue documenting data on adverse events and DAAs, as DAA regimens are a novel concept and require continued monitoring.

12.1 Elbasvir/Grazoprevir

In the C-WORTHY study looking at Genotype 1 patients, both with and without cirrhosis, Elbasvir/Grazoprevir commonly cause asthenia (14%), fatigue (26%), and headache (23%). However, serious events were far less common, occurring in only 3% of patients [27].

12.2 Glecaprevir/Pibrentasvir

The EXPEDITION-1 study evaluated Glecaprevir/Pibrentasvir in compensated cirrhosis across all genotypes except for Genotype 3 and noted that adverse events occurred in 69% of patients, most commonly fatigue and headaches. Severe adverse reactions occurred in 8% of patients, but there was no evidence of a direct drug-induced adverse event [28]. In Genotype 3 patients, either with cirrhosis or prior treatment history, treatment with Glecaprevir/Pibrentasvir was well tolerated with no serious adverse event attributable to the regimen; nor any discontinuations because of an adverse drug reaction [34].

12.3 Ledipasvir/Sofosbuvir

ION-1 examined Genotype 1 patients without cirrhosis and in patients with compensated cirrhosis. Fatigue, headache, insomnia, and nausea were commonly observed adverse events. However, the overall safety profile was excellent, with no patients discontinuing the study due to adverse events [30]. Another study involving Genotype 4 patients, both with compensated cirrhosis and no history of cirrhosis also showed that Ledipasvir/Sofosbuvir is well-tolerated, with no serious adverse events and no discontinuations noted [37]. Genotype 5 patients receiving Ledipasvir/Sofosbuvir commonly had mild symptoms including asthenia, fatigue, and headache. One patient had a serious adverse reaction, but that was judged to be unrelated to DAA therapy [38].

12.4 Sofosbuvir/Daclatasvir

The ALLY-1 trial involved the use of sofosbuvir/daclatasvir and ribavirin in patients with advanced cirrhosis across all major genotypes. Few serious adverse events were noted in the study, none of which could be directly attributable as a consequence of a drug. Anemia is a common side effect of ribavirin [42].

12.5 Sofosbuvir/Velpatasvir

A large study involving genotypes 1, 2, 4, 5,6 and patients with both compensated cirrhosis and no history of cirrhosis showed a good safety profile. Less than 1% of patients discontinued therapy due to adverse reactions. There was no significant difference between the placebo group and the experimental group when it came to adverse events. The most common adverse events noted were fatigue, headache, nasopharyngitis, and nausea [31]. Another study examining Genotype 3 infections, 2% of patients had adverse events severe enough to cause discontinuation. Common adverse events were fatigue, headache, insomnia, and nausea [35].

13. Summary

Direct-acting antivirals represent a breakthrough in the treatment of hepatitis C virus. It has the potential to reduce the global burden of disease caused by the natural hepatitis C history, including cirrhosis, decompensation, and hepatocellular carcinoma. It may also reduce the economic burden of liver transplants. The patient's with existing compensated cirrhosis remain at an elevated risk of numerous other complications, so it is imperative to have an appropriate therapy to help mitigate poor patient outcomes. There are numerous options with the new DAA and being able to appropriately select a regimen will allow for optimal sustained virologic responses in patients with compensated cirrhosis. The AASLD guidelines provide an excellent tool to help dictate a therapy which is tailored to each patient and genotype. As more research is collected on this novel therapy, DAA regimens have the potential to improve on its already remarkable efficacy.

Conflict of interest

None.

Author details

Vijay Gayam[1*], Arshpal Gill[2], Pavani Garlapati[1] and Smruti Mohanty[3]

1 Department of Medicine and Gastroenterology, Interfaith Medical Center, Brooklyn, NY, United States

2 American University of Antigua School of Medicine, Coolidge, Barbuda

3 Department of Medicine and Division of Gastroenterology and Hepatology, New York-Presbyterian Brooklyn Methodist Hospital, Brooklyn, NY, United States

*Address all correspondence to: vgayam@interfaithmedical.com

References

[1] Lingala S, Ghany MG. Natural history of hepatitis C. Gastroenterology Clinics. 2015;**44**(4):717-734

[2] Webster DP, Klenerman P, Dusheiko GM. Hepatitis C. Lancet. 2015;**385**(9973):1124-1135

[3] Manns M, Wedemeyer H, Cornberg M. Treating viral hepatitis C: Efficacy, side effects, and complications. Gut. 2006;**55**(9):1350-1359

[4] Lin J et al. Virus-related liver cirrhosis: Molecular basis and therapeutic options. World Journal of Gastroenterology: WJG. 2014;**20**(21):6457

[5] Westbrook RH, Dusheiko G. Natural history of hepatitis C. Journal of Hepatology. 2014;**61**(1):S58-S68

[6] Pradat P, Virlogeux V, Trépo E. Epidemiology and elimination of HCV-related liver disease. Viruses. 2018;**10**(10):545

[7] Tampaki M, Savvanis S, Koskinas J. Impact of direct-acting antiviral agents on the development of hepatocellular carcinoma: Evidence and pathophysiological issues. Annals of Gastroenterology. 2018;**31**(6):670

[8] Syed T et al. Hepatocellular carcinoma occurrence and recurrence in hepatitis C-infected patients treated with direct-acting antivirals. Cureus. 2018;**10**(6)

[9] Kuftinec G et al. De novo hepatocellular carcinoma occurrence in hepatitis C cirrhotics treated with direct-acting antiviral agents. Hepatic Oncology. 2018;**5**(01):HEP06

[10] Conti F et al. Early occurrence and recurrence of hepatocellular carcinoma in HCV-related cirrhosis treated with direct-acting antivirals. Journal of Hepatology. 2016;**65**(4):727-733

[11] Ferrarese A et al. Hepatitis C virus related cirrhosis decreased as indication to liver transplantation since the introduction of direct-acting antivirals: A single-center study. World Journal of Gastroenterology. 2018;**24**(38):4403

[12] Kieran JA et al. Hepatitis C in the era of direct-acting antivirals: Real-world costs of untreated chronic hepatitis C; a cross-sectional study. BMC Infectious Diseases. 2015;**15**(1):471

[13] Itokawa N et al. Efficacy of direct-acting antiviral treatment in patients with compensated liver cirrhosis: A multicenter study. Hepatology Research. 2018

[14] Chae HB, Park SM, Youn SJ. Direct-acting antivirals for the treatment of chronic hepatitis C: Open issues and future perspectives. The Scientific World Journal. 2013;**2013**: Article ID 704912, 9 pages

[15] Ahmed A, Felmlee D. Mechanisms of hepatitis C viral resistance to direct acting antivirals. Viruses. 2015;**7**(12):6716-6729

[16] Hepatitis C guidelines: AASLD-IDSA recommendations for testing, managing, and treating adults infected with hepatitis C virus. www.hcvguidelines.org

[17] Enomoto M et al. Short-term histological evaluations after achieving a sustained virologic response to direct-acting antiviral treatment for chronic hepatitis C. United European Gastroenterology Journal. 2018;**6**(9):1391-1400

[18] Ansaldi F et al. Hepatitis C virus in the new era: Perspectives in epidemiology, prevention, diagnostics

and predictors of response to therapy. World Journal of Gastroenterology: WJG. 2014;**20**(29):9633

[19] Douglass CH et al. Pathways to ensure universal and affordable access to hepatitis C treatment. BMC Medicine. 2018;**16**(1):175

[20] Cipriano LE, Goldhaber-Fiebert JD. Population health and cost-effectiveness implications of a "treat all" recommendation for HCV: A review of the model-based evidence. MDM Policy & Practice. 2018;**3**(1):2381468318776634

[21] Hui L. Quantifying the effects of aging and urbanization on major gastrointestinal diseases to guide preventative strategies. BMC Gastroenterology. 2018;**18**(1):145

[22] van de Ven N et al. Minimum target prices for production of direct-acting antivirals and associated diagnostics to combat hepatitis C virus. Hepatology. 2015;**61**(4):1174-1182

[23] Colombo M, Lleo A. The impact of antiviral therapy on hepatocellular carcinoma epidemiology. Hepatic Oncology. 2018;**5**(01):HEP03

[24] Majumdar A, Kitson M, Roberts S. Systematic review: Current concepts and challenges for the direct-acting antiviral era in hepatitis C cirrhosis. Alimentary Pharmacology & Therapeutics. 2016;**43**(12):1276-1292

[25] Messina JP et al. Global distribution and prevalence of hepatitis C virus genotypes. Hepatology. 2015;**61**(1):77-87

[26] Gayam V et al. Sofosbuvir based regimens in the treatment of chronic hepatitis C with compensated liver cirrhosis in community care setting. International Journal of Hepatology. 2018;**2018**: Article ID 4136253, 8 pages

[27] Lawitz E et al. Efficacy and safety of 12 weeks versus 18 weeks of treatment with grazoprevir (MK-5172) and elbasvir (MK-8742) with or without ribavirin for hepatitis C virus genotype 1 infection in previously untreated patients with cirrhosis and patients with previous null response with or without cirrhosis (C-WORTHY): A randomised, open-label phase 2 trial. The Lancet. 2015;**385**(9973):1075-1086

[28] Forns X et al. Glecaprevir plus pibrentasvir for chronic hepatitis C virus genotype 1, 2, 4, 5, or 6 infection in adults with compensated cirrhosis (EXPEDITION-1): A single-arm, open-label, multicentre phase 3 trial. The Lancet Infectious Diseases. 2017;**17**(10):1062-1068

[29] Chayama K et al. Efficacy and safety of glecaprevir/pibrentasvir in Japanese patients with chronic genotype 1 hepatitis C virus infection with and without cirrhosis. Journal of Gastroenterology. 2018;**53**(4):557-565

[30] Afdhal N et al. Ledipasvir and sofosbuvir for untreated HCV genotype 1 infection. New England Journal of Medicine. 2014;**370**(20):1889-1898

[31] Feld JJ et al. Sofosbuvir and velpatasvir for HCV genotype 1, 2, 4, 5, and 6 infection. New England Journal of Medicine. 2015;**373**(27):2599-2607

[32] Toyoda H et al. Efficacy and safety of glecaprevir/pibrentasvir in Japanese patients with chronic genotype 2 hepatitis C virus infection. Hepatology. 2018;**67**(2):505-513

[33] Nelson D et al. P0782: All-oral 12-week combination treatment with daclatasvir (DCV) and sofosbuvir (SOF) in treatment-experienced patients infected with HCV genotype (GT) 3: A subanalysis of the ALLY-3 phase 3 study. Journal of Hepatology. 2015;**62**:S624

[34] Wyles D et al. Glecaprevir/pibrentasvir for hepatitis C virus genotype 3 patients with cirrhosis and/or prior treatment experience: A partially randomized phase 3 clinical trial. Hepatology. 2018;**67**(2):514-523

[35] Foster GR et al. Sofosbuvir and velpatasvir for HCV genotype 2 and 3 infection. New England Journal of Medicine. 2015;**373**(27):2608-2617

[36] Gayam V et al. Direct-acting antivirals in chronic hepatitis C genotype 4 infection in community care setting. Gastroenterology Research. 2018;**11**(2):130

[37] Kohli A et al. Ledipasvir and sofosbuvir for hepatitis C genotype 4: A proof-of-concept, single-Centre, open-label phase 2a cohort study. The Lancet Infectious Diseases. 2015;**15**(9):1049-1054

[38] Abergel A et al. Ledipasvir-sofosbuvir in patients with hepatitis C virus genotype 5 infection: An open-label, multicentre, single-arm, phase 2 study. The Lancet Infectious Diseases. 2016;**16**(4):459-464

[39] Planas R et al. Natural history of decompensated hepatitis C virus-related cirrhosis. A study of 200 patients. Journal of Hepatology. 2004;**40**(5):823-830

[40] Tsai J et al. Effect of hepatitis C and B virus infection on risk of hepatocellular carcinoma: A prospective study. British Journal of Cancer. 1997;**76**(7):968

[41] Everson GT. Treatment of chronic hepatitis C in patients with decompensated cirrhosis. Reviews in Gastroenterological Disorders. 2004;**4**:S31-S38

[42] Poordad F et al. Daclatasvir with sofosbuvir and ribavirin for hepatitis C virus infection with advanced cirrhosis or post-liver transplantation recurrence. Hepatology. 2016;**63**(5):1493-1505

[43] Curry MP et al. Sofosbuvir and velpatasvir for HCV in patients with decompensated cirrhosis. New England Journal of Medicine. 2015;**373**(27):2618-2628

[44] Toshikuni N, Arisawa T, Tsutsumi M. Hepatitis C-related liver cirrhosis-strategies for the prevention of hepatic decompensation, hepatocarcinogenesis, and mortality. World Journal of Gastroenterology: WJG. 2014;**20**(11):2876

[45] Kaczmarek DJ et al. Alterations of the NK cell pool in HIV/HCV co-infection. PLoS One. 2017;**12**(4):e0174465

[46] Bräu N et al. Treatment of chronic hepatitis C in HIV/HCV-coinfection with interferon α-2b+ full-course vs. 16-week delayed ribavirin. Hepatology. 2004;**39**(4):989-998

[47] Wyles DL et al. Daclatasvir plus sofosbuvir for HCV in patients coinfected with HIV-1. New England Journal of Medicine. 2015;**373**(8):714-725

[48] Gayam V et al. Real-world clinical efficacy and tolerability of direct-acting antivirals in hepatitis C monoinfection compared to hepatitis C/human immunodeficiency virus coinfection in a community care setting. Gut and Liver. 2018;**12**(6):694-703

[49] Denniston MM et al. Chronic hepatitis C virus infection in the United States, national health and nutrition examination survey 2003 to 2010. Annals of Internal Medicine. 2014;**160**(5):293-300

[50] Reddy KR et al. Racial differences in responses to therapy with interferon in chronic hepatitis C. Hepatology. 1999;**30**(3):787-793

[51] Gayam V et al. Sofosbuvir based regimens in the treatment of chronic hepatitis C genotype 1 infection in African–American patients: A community-based retrospective cohort study. European Journal of Gastroenterology & Hepatology. 2018;**30**(10):1200

[52] Wilder JM et al. Safety and efficacy of ledipasvir-sofosbuvir in black patients with hepatitis C virus infection: A retrospective analysis of phase 3 data. Hepatology. 2016;**63**(2):437-444

[53] Putz-Bankuti C et al. Association of 25-hydroxyvitamin D levels with liver dysfunction and mortality in chronic liver disease. Liver International. 2012;**32**(5):845-851

[54] Lange CM et al. Genetic analyses reveal a role for vitamin D insufficiency in HCV-associated hepatocellular carcinoma development. PLoS One. 2013;**8**(5):e64053

[55] Gayam V et al. Association between vitamin D levels and treatment response to direct-acting antivirals in chronic hepatitis C: A real-world study. Gastroenterology Research. 2018;**11**(4):309

[56] Bourlière M et al. Sofosbuvir, velpatasvir, and voxilaprevir for previously treated HCV infection. New England Journal of Medicine. 2017;**376**(22):2134-2146